THE HEALING POWER
OF HERBS

by

May Bethel

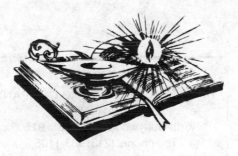

Published by
Melvin Powers
WILSHIRE BOOK COMPANY
12015 Sherman Road
No. Hollywood, California 91605
Telephone: (213) 875-1711

First Published July 1968

© May Bethel 1968

I dedicate this book to my family, who
encouraged my study of herbs and
foods in the prevention and treatment
of disease.

Printed by

HAL LEIGHTON PRINTING COMPANY
P.O. Box 3952
North Hollywood, California 91605
Telephone: (213) 983-1105

Printed in the United States of America
ISBN 0-87980-047-X

Contents

CHAPTER I

A History of Herbalism

THE knowledge of the use of herbs in the prevention and treatment of disease is a lost art. The use of herbs goes back to the beginning of time.

A systematic study of plant life probably first began among the ancient Egyptians and Greeks.

Hippocrates was the first man who practised medicine as an art. He was a Greek physician who lived about the fourth century before Christ. In his writings, Hippocrates described plants as medicine. He was a herbal practitioner.

The following is taken from Pliny's *Natural History*, written almost 2,000 years ago. "Hippocrates verely had this honour above all men, that hee was the first who wrote with most perspicuitic of Physicke, and reduced the precepts and rules thereof into the bodle of an art; howbeit, in all his books we find no other recipes but herbs."

Those who followed Hippocrates made a more systematic study and classification of plants and their uses as medicine. The best of these herbals or books describing wild and cultivated plants was written by Otto Brunfels, a German botanist. His contemporary, Hieronymous Bock, produced the *Materia Medica*.

Herbs were used as medicine extensively until about 1500 when Hohemhein started the practice of using chemicals to treat disease. Medical men then followed the idea that the human body could be purified chemically. He, Hohemhein, publicly burned the books of Hippocrates and Galen, another herbalist. He transformed the medical practice. After his death (Hohemhein's), hundreds of people took up the practice of giving chemicals in place of herbs, roots and barks. He was the first to give mercury as a medicine.

The herbalists of Great Britain are the true successors of Galen and Hippocrates. Those of the medical profession today are the successors of the descendants of Hohemhein of the fifteenth century.

The American Indians had a knowledge of many herbs, roots and barks and their use in the treating of disease. Many of these wild plants helped them keep vigorous in spite of their rigorous existence. As a result, they had great stamina and endurance.

Squaws served as domestics in colonial homes. They often used their native medicines in the care of the sick and taught their white employers their herbal knowledge.

Native plants were the sole source of medicine for the early pioneers of America.

A century ago most American housewives were acquainted with the medicinal properties of herbs. Young girls were taken into the fields by their mothers, who taught them to recognize many herbs and to know their use in treating disease.

CHAPTER II

What Herbs Can Do

THE knowledge and use of herbs should be challenging to every thinking person who is concerned about his health and the health of his family.

God has provided a remedy for every disease that might afflict man. Every part of the world has its herbs which are peculiar to that particular area, to be used with wisdom in treating disease.

Chemical wonder-drugs are not the answer to our need. For no drug is ever free from side-effects.

Botanicals were created for a purpose, and that purpose should be as clearly understood by us today as it was by the colonists and the Indians who they found here.

It has been said that knowledge is power and he who seeks it is wise, and he who neglects it does so to his own regret.

The fundamental principle of natural healing calls for a return to organic remedies.

We may complain about the weeds that clutter our gardens and fence-corners, but weeds are herbs which we have not yet learned to identify and cultivate.

The Office of Indian Affairs sent a group of specialists to visit the Navajo Indians to prove the superiority of modern medical methods. They reported that the ancient methods used by the Indian doctors proved as fully effective in curing many diseases as had the latest methods known to medical science.

No one herb can be said to cure any ailment. Each element working together in the correct proportion to each other helps nature in her healing and rejuvenating process. A combination of herbs is better, since all the minerals will then be contained in the tea and a perfect balance will be more nearly certain.

Research is substantiating the truths herbalists have known

for centuries. Schools of Pharmacy are granted enormous sums to study the relation of plant chemistry to the restoration of health and resistance to disease.

However, it must be stressed again that the alkaloids chemically produced from a plant are not as effective as the tea from the original plant.

Only with herbs can the desired results be obtained, since in them there are properties as yet unidentified which also are essential to proper body maintenance.

Our bodies are equipped with everything necessary to prevent illness and disease.

Experiments have proved that the process known as metabolism, that is, the breaking down and the building up of cells, is kept in perfect harmony with the consumption of plants and plant juices such as herb teas and vegetable juices. This vegetable matter has a distinct influence on gland activity and therefore restores health to afflicted parts of the body. Since the body cannot retain these essential elements, it is necessary to provide them every day.

The body has recuperative powers. But don't expect miracles overnight. Nature sometimes works slowly. Illness does not happen overnight, either. You cannot side-step nature's laws and escape illness and disease. You cannot go on for months and years ignoring nature's laws and expect miracles after you reach a point of no return.

Since most botanicals are mild, we must work with nature to obtain the best results. Detrimental habits can hinder inherent healing powers. Avoid tobacco, coffee, tea and liquor. Diet should consist of mineral and vitamin rich foods of easy digestion.

Herbs that are specific for particular ailments require certain amounts. You may have heard it said that "If a little will do good, a lot'll do better". This is a serious mistake. Large amounts of herb teas can be toxic and dangerous. No more so though than being gluttonous in eating foods of any kind.

Health is the complete absence of disease. A healthy body is the surest safeguard against any form of disease.

If a deadly fungus is swallowed, a healthy reaction is a

vigorous and complete emptying of the stomach and bowels. The better the health, the more decisive will this house-cleaning be. The more thorough and immediate the evacuation, the less damage will be done to organs and tissues. To stop this method of nature would be dangerous. Herb teas will assist nature in throwing off these poisons while chemically produced medicine might cause these symptoms to abate, which is a common practice.

Out of the man's trouser leg fell a shining ant as big as a scorpion and with a long sting at its tail. It had an extremely hard skull. It was almost impossible to crush it. This incident occurred in the tropics where such insects are found. A native said, "The little brute is worse than a scorpion, but it isn't dangerous to a healthy man."

If man would resort to simple means, follow simple laws of health, nature would restore the body to normal health and protect it against outside hazards.

Herbs have scientific basis. A noted German scientist and author, W. Weitzel, in his book *The Mysteries of Plant Blood*, illustrated how plant blood (juices) and human blood are closely associated and that roots, barks and herbs have value in building up health and resistance to disease.

Simple cures are not enough for medical science. For most every "cure" brought about by herbs, there is a so called expert who says such a cure is merely a coincidence.

However, herbs can be an effective agent in disease prevention as well as assisting nature in her healing process.

Everyone should have a knowledge of what herbs can do.

Herb remedies or folk remedies and folk-lore are associated together, which is a mistake. Folk-lore can be amusing in its superstitions in the care of the sick. On the other hand, folk medicine or herbalism is rich in herbal wisdom. If we would use herbs, we would be doing our bodies a favour.

Modern chemistry can isolate substances from plants. However, after fifty years or more it has been established that the original herb tea, containing all the principles necessary to healing, is far more effective than the isolated principles or alkaloids.

Modern medicines are complex, powerful agents. A person's insides are literally pickled in chemicals. Medicants today squeeze out of the coal-tar barrel every available bit of harm to afflicted man.

Plant drugs have stood the test of time far longer than the scalpel, antibiotics and vaccines.

A lack of knowledge based on truth is accountable for much of the suffering and misery of humanity. A practical knowledge of the use of herbs would save money, suffering and often premature death.

In Ecclesiastes we find these words, "The Lord created medicines out of the earth and a wise man will not abhor them."

CHAPTER III

Doctor or Drug Induced Disease

In the December 31, 1963, issue of *Look* magazine it was reported that at least 10% of all medical patients are suffering from diseases caused by their doctors.

At Johns Hopkins Hospital in Baltimore, Maryland, it was estimated that the actual number of Americans who are made sick yearly by the treatment of their doctors is 1,300,000. Of this number many thousands die, killed by improper medical treatment administered by licensed doctors, whose knowledge is so inadequate that 80% of the time they are not certain of what is wrong with their patients. In their uncertainty they blindly prescribe potent drugs.

Medical schools are staffed with scientists and specialists, most of whom never practised medicine. They teach more and more of scientific quackery and less and less sound, practical medical knowledge. The most dangerous men are those with a medical education who have never practised medicine.

It is shocking to see the ease with which potent drugs are adopted by medical practitioners. Surveys show that many doctors rely heavily, if not exclusively, on the recommendations in advertisements in medical journals. It is appalling how many doctors take the facts in pharmaceutical advertisements as gospel truth without looking into the possible harmful effects of the drugs they administer.

Many iatrogenic diseases can be traced to new drugs with potent side-effects.

Iatrogenic is a word coined by the doctors themselves. Iatro is a Greek word meaning "a doctor". Genic means "caused by".

The list of iatrogenic disorders runs into the thousands and grows longer every day, which proves a popular aphorism that the remedy is worse than the disease.

Potent drugs have definite side-effects. An AMA study group admitted that there is always a calculated risk in administering drugs to a patient. For example, they have been warned against the use of chloromycetin, which seems to have a definite toxic action on the bone marrow where the blood cells are produced.

New drugs present greater potential danger than ever before. They are promoted by aggressive sales campaigns that overstate their merits and fail to indicate the risks involved by their use. More than 20% of the drugs listed since 1956 in the publication *New and Non-official Drugs* were found worthless or potentially dangerous.

According to the May 1962 issue of *Consumer Reports*, a pharmaceutical company puts a drug on the market and is withdrawn from the market only after it seriously injures numbers of people or proves fatal.

Much of the public is unaware of the dangerous side-effects of the potent drugs administered by our doctors.

Are we becoming a drugged generation?

Why is it the average person will be especially careful in buying a suit of clothes, even checking the fibres to see if it is made of good material or some shoddy stuff, and yet blindly accept a tablet or other medication without a thought as to its medicinal merits? Or allows a serum to be injected into his bloodstream without questioning its merit or even harm?

Dr. Bostock (author *The History of Medicine*) says that every dose of medicine given is a blind experiment upon the vitality of a patient.

Dr. Schweniger, a physician to the Prince of Bismarck, said that people want to be cheated. They think that no cure is possible without medicine. He says that doctors have been talking "this apothecary stuff" to them until they believe it.

Hippocrates knew that nature did the real curing. He recognized that the prime physician in any case is nature. The doctor's role should be to work with nature. A doctor's job is more important than just curing sick folks. He should also try to keep healthy folks healthy.

Dr. Julia B. Mackenzie and Dr. C. G. Mackenzie, of the

Johns Hopkins School of Hygiene, found that sulpha drugs can cause thyroid enlargement. It is also known that the sulphas can injure the kidneys.

Dr. Sam C. Little, of the University of Michigan Medical School, reported that all members of the sulpha drug family have a poisonous effect on the nervous system.

Sulpha and the antibiotics also affect the nutrition. They discourage the growth of valuable bacteria. Without a good culture in the intestines, you can expect trouble.

Dr. Irving H. Itkin, head of allergy and asthma research at the National Jewish Hospital in Denver, Colorado, told the Associated Press that the use of antibiotics and steroid drugs kill off the lactobacillus acidophilus and other benign bacteria which normally destroy harmful bacteria.

Indiscriminate dosing with the anti-histamines has produced disastrous results. They can affect the nervous system, the heart and the digestive tract.

In *JAMA*, February 3, 1951, is a report that overdoses of anti-histamine caused the death of eleven persons, eight of them children. Dr. J. B. Wyngarden in *JAMA* (vol. 145, p. 277) disclosed that common reaction to anti-histamine includes drowsiness, dizziness, headache, insomnia, nervousness, vomiting, constipation and diarrhoea. It may also cause a grave blood disease, agranulocytosis.

Tranquillizers are a chemical substance which affects the central nervous system, reducing anxiety and tension and allowing the individual to become relaxed and calm. Tranquillizers have such names as miltown, equanil, compazine, thorazine, sparine, serpasil and librium. Most of these are derivatives of one or two drugs; chlorpromazine, a synthetic product discovered by French chemists, and resperine, a natural chemical found in the juices of an Indian shrub called snakeroot or Rauwolfia serpentina. Tranquillizers are used to relax mental patients.

One of the most used drugs to quiet restlessness and induce sleep is barbital. Like other powerful drugs, barbiturates may be purchased by anybody, any time and anywhere. Constant use causes slow poisoning. Illnesses and injuries become fatal

B

by lowered resistance from the use of barbiturates over an extended period. A combination of alcohol and barbiturates is more violent than twice the amount of either taken alone.

Tranquillizers taken to treat high blood pressure trigger depressions serious enough to send some persons to the hospital for psychiatric care. This report was given by Dr. Robert L. Faucett, of the Mayo Clinic of Rochester, Minnesota, to the American Psychiatric Association.

The major tranquilizers chlorpromazine and resperine are extremely potent and should definitely not be used for occasional anxiety.

Tranquillizers may also cause hepatitis and tremors similar to Parkinson's disease. White blood count may also fall dangerously and motor co-ordination may be affected. They have also been known to cause loss of hearing and serious liver troubles.

Doctors still are not agreed on how they work or how long to treat with tranquillizers or their long-range effects, yet they are used promiscuously. Tranquillizers are the pharmaceutical bonanza of this generation.

Dr. Paul Dudley White, the famous heart specialist, says, "Out of the window with those tranquillizer pills and out of the door yourself for a good brisk walk." Walking is the best tranquillizer of all.

A reader objected to a full-page advertisement in a medical journal which suggested using a tranquillizer to treat hyperactive children. An active child is a healthy child. Could anyone be so foolish as to use these potentially dangerous drugs to quiet an active healthy child?

Mer/29, a product of the William S. Merrill Company, a drug intended for reducing blood cholesterol, was found to cause cataracts, baldness and changes in hair and skin colour. It was on the market for two years before it was finally withdrawn, after it was taken by more than 300,000 people. Clinical information such as this was available before the end of 1961, yet Mer/29, or triparanol, was still manufactured and sold to doctors who continued to prescribe it. The purpose of this drug is to lower body cholesterol by inhibiting its being made by the body, which in itself is dangerous. No interference should ever be made with the body's own ability to produce cholesterol. The Press and TV have made people cholesterol conscious.

The drug dinitrophenol, much used in treating obesity, has been found to cause cataracts.

According to Dr. Walter Modell, head physician of the Department of Clinical Pharmacology of Cornell University Medical School, the effectiveness of anti-coagulants has been questioned. In spite of the fact that there is serious doubt as to their effectiveness, doctors still continue to prescribe these dangerous drugs.

Certain anti-hypertension drugs, especially the Rauwolfia derivatives and phenothiazine compound, in combination with certain anesthetics, can cause severe low blood presure.

The court at Buffalo, New York, approved a settlement of $3,100 against the Eli Lilly and Company, manufacturers of the drug ilotycin, and McKesson and Robbins, distributors. One hundred mgs of the drug was injected into a 10-year-old girl after a tonsillectomy. She was unable to walk for five months after the injection.

Ilosone is known to have caused liver injury and jaundice. Neomycin has caused deafness. Impairment of hearing and dizziness may be due to excessive dosage of streptomycin. Serious allergic reactions have been brought about by the use of penicillin.

In *Anti-biotics and Chemotherapy* (March 1962) an article by Dr. Murray Robinson points out that Ilosone, a drug commonly used to treat staphylococcus infection, caused liver poisoning in fifteen out of ninety-three patients.

Hydralazine, used in treating high blood pressure, has been known to produce angina pectoris in some cases.

Even though there is careful planning of antibiotic therapy, post-surgical antibiotics have been found to be useless. Doctors know how they work and what their limitations are and yet they continue their use.

Cortisone, a drug much used to treat arthritis, also has serious side-effects.

Cortisones are drugs modelled after the hormones produced by the adrenal cortex, the outer part of the adrenal gland.

The list of side-effects of cortisone lengthens day by day. In *Science New Letter* for December 1, 1962, was a warning about prolonged or large doses of cortisone.

A report in *JAMA* tells about sixteen patients who were treated for arthritis and two with chronic bronchial asthma, got cataracts after long-term use of corticosteroids.

A doctor whose letter appeared in *The Digest of Treatment* for October 1951, attributed the suicide of one of his patients to cortisone treatments.

In *Modern Medicine* for May 1954 an article pointed out that within a few hours after cortisone therapy begins, the patient feels restless and irritable and that emotional instability follows.

In *Chemical Week* for January 26, 1957, was a warning by the Federal Drug Administration against over-the-counter sales of corticosteroids, yet one of the large drug companies in their publication advocated self-injection with cortisone as a practical and effective mode of treatment in severe rheumatoid arthritis over long periods.

The damage to bones that results in easy fracture has been reported after cortisone therapy. In the *JAMA* for October 2, 1954, is a report of multiple fracture of the spine in four patients receiving cortisone. The *Lancet* for June 1, 1957, affirms the fact that steroids can be a direct cause of death.

When the corticosteroids first appeared, their potential sounded like a panacea for all the illness of man. Now after ten years of experience with the dangerous side-effects of these drugs, they are still high on the list of popular treatments.

Scientists have been studying interferon, a new versatile substance that may be able to protect the body against colds, 'flu, polio, smallpox, cancer, etc. The body manufactures interferon as a defence against disease. It must be produced in sufficient amounts. The researchers idea is to keep the body's normal interferon response at full strength. Just how they expect to do this is still a question for research and possibly more drugs to do the job.

The body's ability to protect itself (manufacture interferon) against toxins, viruses, bacteria and other causes of illness is seriously hampered by taking aspirin.

Dr. Alexander Langmuir, chief of the epidemiology section of the Communicable Disease Center pointed out that the widespread use of vaccines among the general population cannot be justified.

The *Phoenix Arizona Republic* of November 1963 quotes Dr. Raymond Reed, an Arizona veterinarian, as saying that the incidence of paralysis as a side-effect from the use of the Pasteur anti-rabies vaccine is about as high as the chance of exposure to rabies from dog bite. He also says that if an animal bites through clothing and has a dry mouth, the chance of actual exposure to rabies is very slight.

When bitten by strange dogs, people are prone to insist on immediate innoculation with anti-rabies vaccine. It should be certain that the dog was really rabid. This or any injection should not be given without sufficient cause.

The Food and Drug Administration is sworn to protect the American public. However, according to Dr. John Nestor, it gives more protection to the interests of the large drug companies and the pharmaceutical houses.

Dr. Nestor, a 50-year-old pediatric and cardiology specialist in the division of the FDA that deals with drugs, gave investigators details of a number of cases to back his contention that the FDA has decided cases in favour of the pharmaceutical houses.

Testimony has been given that drugs are allowed to remain on the market for months after the FDA doctors declare that neither the safety nor the efficacy of the drugs has been proven.

Dr. Nestor also charged that non-medical men, including laymen, have made medical decisions.

Committee chairman Hubert Humphrey, and Senator Ernest Gruening, of Alaska, call the situation shocking. Humphrey is a former pharmacist. He told in his report that drugs intended for use by victims of chronic diseases were released by FDA even before chronic toxicity tests were completed on animals. Also that reports of injuries and deaths to test patients received by drug companies have not been reported to FDA or have been skilfully withheld. Drugs have been approved that FDA now admits should never have been approved.

In 1963, Estes Kefauver opened a compaign for lowering drug prices. In his bill the senator said, "A price which is more than five times the cost of production (including an appropriate allowance for research) is excessive."

Approximately one billion dollars was allocated in 1964 to the numerous health societies. Much of this money is spent for advertising under the guise of "Public Education". Misleading and often false statements are made. The medical profession spends more money advertising than does any other health profession. Big business has assumed the role of medical adviser.

High-pressured advertising stampeded people into using wonder-drugs. False scare-advertising gives false hope. This is also true where vaccines and shots are concerned.

Dr. Charles E. Page, of Boston, said that he had been a regular practitioner of medicine in Boston for thirty-three years. Also that he had studied the question of vaccination earnestly for forty-five years. He said that as for vaccination as a preventive of disease, there is not a scrap of evidence in its favour. He also said that injection of serum into the bloodstream does not prevent smallpox. We also hear of failures of polio vaccines.

Quoting Hippocrates, "Leave your drugs in the chemist's pot if you cannot heal the patient with food." Hippocrates also said, "He who for an ordinary cause resigns the fate of his patient to mercury (chemicals) is a vile enemy to the sick."

An alarming series of car accidents have been traced to the side-effects of modern drugs. Few people outside of the medical and pharmaceutical professions know how deadly our modern drugs really are. Anti-histamine, taken for colds, act like a knockout drug. Such drugs affect the vision, bring on drowsiness, make reaction time and mental processes sluggish. Such symptoms may come on swiftly. If you become jittery or develop an overpowering urge to sleep, don't drive.

Dr. Walter Modell is of the opinion that it is highly improbable that a drug will ever be produced which has no side-effects.

One doctor said that any warning from the medical profession would only prevent some people from taking the medicine at all.

What the medical profession is searching for is better drugs, better surgical procedures, better vaccines and serums. They are not searching for prevention.

Can you imagine a world of laboratory specimens, fed with chemicals and repaired with the mechanics of surgery?

I hope I have stimulated your thinking. Many need to be blasted out of their complacency.

Doctor or drug induced disease is something to be feared.

CHAPTER IV

Herbal Treatment of Disease

NATURE has the intrinsic ability to regenerate itself. However, when nature needs help, turn to herbs.

AGUE

For ague, also called intermittent fever, gentian, sorrel, tansy, vervain, camomile are the recommended herbs.

ANAEMIA

In anaemia there is a low state of the blood. The number of red corpuscles is decreased.

One hears of iron-deficiency anaemia. Iron alone cannot help anaemia. It has been found that if the diet is deficient in vitamin C long enough, anaemia will result. Iron needs vitamin C in its process of absorption. Along with an iron and vitamin C deficiency, a deficiency in copper, manganese, cobalt and magnesium can cause anaemia. These minerals are especially necessary in haemoglobin formation.

Synthetic vitamin C is not effective in treating anaemia. Only natural vitamin C as found in rosehips, containing other factors necessary to the effective functioning of vitamin C, is useful in treating anaemia as well as other vitamin C deficiency diseases.

Alterative botanicals were long used in cases of impoverished blood. Alterative is an obsolete term also called blood purifiers. What they really do is restore to the body such elements as are necessary to a healthy bloodstream. A healthy bloodstream largely determines the power of resistance to disease. Botanic alteratives contain a variety of ingredients known today as trace minerals which are not always found in the foods we eat.

A combination of Rocky Mountain grape root, butternut bark and marshmallow root is a good alterative. Alterative botanicals long used in cases of impoverished blood are dandelion root, yellow dock root, yarrow, wild cherry bark, comfrey and red raspberry leaves.

Black walnut leaves are especially good to restore the red corpuscles and iron compounds. They are the best blood builders. The green pigment in the leaves (chlorophyll) is rich in iron. Chlorophyll is similar chemically to the non-protein portion of haemoglobin.

APPENDICITIS

Constipation is one of the causes of appendicitis, which, of course, is due mostly to a faulty diet. In the case of appendicitis, the first thing to do is to give an enema, using either a small amount of baking soda or a herb tea. This will often relieve the pain. For a herbal enema, use either spearmint or catnip. Apply hot and cold packs alternately in the region of the appendix and all along the spine. A poultice of mullein leaves (a large handful), one tablespoon powdered lobelia and a pinch of ginger is good, made by adding enough slippery elm bark (shredded) or cornmeal to the tea to make it thick enough to spread. Apply as warm as patient can stand it and leave it on until cool. After the attack go on a liquid diet of fruit and vegetable juices and alkaline broths. A calmative tea is also good. Never give solid food, water or a laxative during an attack. These helps are good while waiting for the doctor, but always see your practitioner.

ARTHRITIS

Arthritis is an inflammation of the connective tissue in the joints. Pain is not the disease itself. It is the result of a long-standing nutritional imbalance.

Our modern, improper diets and stresses encourage the formation of toxins in the digestive tract.

At one time teeth, tonsils and appendix were removed because they were thought to be the source of toxins that caused arthritis. However, when arthritics still had their pains and misery after the removal of these supposed offenders, this procedure was abandoned.

As the disease progresses, the involved joints are moved less and less because of the pain. Consequently the surrounding muscles begin to atrophy, resulting in crippling.

While not a fatal disease, arthritis causes the greatest number of disabilities.

Many types of therapy have been tried to cure arthritis. It is admitted though that a cure has not yet been found.

Any factor that adds to the state of health may be considered as helpful.

Be optimistic, be patient and persistent. A pessimistic attitude upsets the whole glandular system, causing functional imbalance.

If you feel stiffness coming on, breathe fast and deep for five minutes.

Walking is good if particular attention is paid to posture and breathing. Briskness and duration depends upon the endurance of the individual. Walk should be stopped at a point just short of fatigue.

Take care of your feet. Ill-fitting shoes can cause joint pain.

Correctly applied massage helps to maintain the tone and circulation in the muscles, the activity of which is inhibited by pain. The greatest drawback to massage therapy is the tendency to overdo it. Too much or prolonged massage can be harmful.

While under a hot shower (as hot as can be borne) massage all the area near the aching joint.

Soak the feet in hot Epsom salts water. Then massage every part of the feet, especially the soles.

Also firmly massage the hands, paying particular attention to the palms.

A bath (soak) in hot Epsom salts water will help to alleviate the pain.

Spinal alignment is also helpful.

Exercise daily. Exercise increases the range of motion in the affected joint, strengthens the muscles moving the joint, prevents deformity.

Arthritics should rest often. Rest does not consist merely of cessation from physical and mental labours. Relaxing the muscles is resting. Five minutes of relaxation out of every hour can minimize pain.

Exercise, rest, relaxation, proper food, vitamin and mineral therapy and B-12 injections will go a long way to reduce the pain and discomfort of arthritis.

Since arthritis is a condition of the joints where the bones or cartilage are either eroded or roughened by calcium deposits, there may be an insufficient supply of phosphorus to maintain a calcium balance. Calcium would then be precipitated into the joints or tissues. Almost any deficiency will depress the metabolism of calcium.

It has been found that arthritics have oil deficiencies. Any good vegetable oil is good to add to the diet. Cod liver oil is especially recommended.

Natural vitamins and minerals are always more effective than the synthetic kind. Molasses provide the much needed iron. There is a sulphur deficiency in the cartilage of joints of arthritics. Sulphur is found in amino acids.

Fruit and vegetable juices have eased joint pains, especially raw carrot juice. Celery is recommended as a preventive of arthritis. It is said that if celery is cooked and eaten freely with a little milk, the excess acids in the system would be neutralized and arthritis would be impossible. Parsley is also recommended. Pour one quart of boiling water over one cup of parsley (firmly packed), both leaves and stems. Steep fifteen minutes. One small glassful daily is said to be helpful. Excellent results have been reported in the use of garlic; also uncooked proteins, such as are found in sesame and sunflower seeds and wheat germ, are recommended.

The arthritic has need of an abundance of pantothenic acid,

B-6 and manganese. These are removed from wheat in the milling of flour.

In an animal experiment, one group which was fed cooked foods, including pasteurized milk, developed joint stiffness. In the other group, given the same diet except that raw chard leaves were added, all joint stiffness disappeared.

The best dietetic therapy includes alfalfa, desiccated liver, brewer's yeast, bone meal, fish-liver oil, lecithin, sesame and sunflower, seeds, B-12, parsley, garlic and molasses.

Refrain from eating white sugar, white flour, saturated fats and pastries.

The following recipe is said to be helpful. Put a whole lemon, peel, pulp, and seeds, in a blender with water and honey. Drink this half an hour before eating breakfast or on an empty stomach. Some have used apple cider vinegar and honey, two teaspoonfuls of each in a glass of water before meals.

Some herbs or formulas are helpful. The following are recommended:

Cayenne (amount, size of a pea) in a glass of milk; or a No. 1 capsule filled with the cayenne may be used. Take the capsule with a glass of milk also.

Comfrey has been given to arthritics with amazing results. It may be used as a tea or eaten raw in salads.

I have used rosemary leaves with excellent results. Drink hot every morning and night.

The Mexican yam has been discovered by modern scientists. The tuber is the source of diosgenin, which yields cortisone and other hormones and steroids used in treating rheumatic diseases.

Willow bark tea has been used by African natives for generations to relieve the pain of rheumatism. The willow bark contains salicin, a pain-killing drug.

The medication most often prescribed today for arthritis is aspirin. Salicylic acid is one of the ingredients of aspirin. Wintergreen leaves contain an abundance of salicylic acid. Wintergreen may be prescribed as taken as the oil of the wintergreen. However, care should be taken as to the amount to be taken. Three or four drops in a glass of water or on a half teaspoonful of sugar is sufficient for a dose. This may be taken three or four times a day, not more than every three or four hours.

Arthritis is one of the afflictions of man that requires a good house-cleaning. A daily fast once a week for several weeks is good. Drink copious amounts of pure water and/or fruit juices during the fast. One kind of juice only to be used during a day. Juice may be diluted.

A few herbal formulae which are recommended for arthritis are:

Poke root, one ounce; prickly ash Bark, one ounce; Black Cohosh, half ounce; and Burdock Root, one ounce.

Virginia snake root, prickly ash bark, burdock root, yarrow and wintergreen leaves.

Wahoo bark, Rocky Mountain grape root, black cohosh and wintergreen leaves.

ASTHMA AND HAY FEVER

Asthma is caused by the system being filled with waste matter and mucous. It is recognized by occasional paroxysms of difficult breathing, lasting from a few hours to several days, coming on at intervals to be followed by remissions, during which the patient breathes with comparative ease.

In the case of asthma, the diet should be plain; only raw fruits and vegetables should be eaten for five or six weeks. Nuts may be allowed. This diet should be continued with the addition of fish, lamb or beef broiled. Carbohydrates, refined products, coffee, tea, cocoa or excessive salt have no place in the diet of an asthmatic patient.

An enema should be given every day for a while to help eliminate waste products of metabolism.

Dr. Livingstone discovered that many asthmatic patients may be completely relieved by a course of training in correct breathing. Using the slant-board has helped some.

A syrup made with honey and the tea made from wild plum bark is the best herbal remedy for asthma.

Equal parts of spikenard, elecampane, comfrey, hoarhound and one teaspoonful lobelia is also good. One tablespoonful taken every half hour is recommended.

A good herb mixture is made with equal parts of wild cherry bark, skullcap, valerian, gentian, calamus and a small amount of lobelia.

Black cohosh, coltsfoot, wild cherry, blue vervain are also recommended.

Mullein leaves, dried and smoked in a pipe or cigarette, has helped in some cases. Spikenard was used by the American Indians in the treatment of asthma and hay fever.

MaHuang was used by the Chinese centuries ago. Ephedrin is a drug being extracted from MaHuang. Mormon Valley herb also contains ephedrin.

An anti-spasmodic tincture has been of value in treating asthma. This tincture may be made as follows: Pour one pint of boiling water over once ounce each of scullcap, Gum myrrh, skunk cabbage, one-half ounce each of black cohosh and Cayenne. Steep one-half hour. Strain and add one pint apple cider vinegar. Bottle for use. One teaspoonful is the recommended dose.

A pillow stuffed with "life everlasting" has helped some people.

It has long been suspected that asthma and hay fever are symptoms of a deficiency in the body of some particular factor rather than being a disease in themselves. The failure of the body to assimilate sufficient potassium may well be the cause of asthmatic difficulties based on faulty functioning of the adrenal glands. The herbs containing potassium are walnut leaves, mistletoe, coltsfoot, mullien, yarrow, comfrey, calamus and fennel seed.

Asthma has been helped by a supplement of calcium, phosphorus and vitamin D.

Honey is said to be a cure for hay fever. According to experimental studies made by William Beaumont, of General Hospital of El Paso, Texas, chewing honeycomb from the region in which the patient lives has helped some. By chewing the wax or eating the honey it is possible to counteract the effect of the pollen. The patient builds up a resistance to the very thing for which he has an intolerance.

The body level of vitamin C is decidedly lower during hay fever attacks.

When hay fever starts, or even before the pollen season, take a glassful of "life everlasting" tea night and morning. Also make a pillow using "life everlasting". A diet of fruit juices (50% raw) gives immediate relief.

Before a cure for asthma or hay fever can be effective, the diet of the patient must be corrected.

BACKACHE

Backache is one of the most prevalent and perhaps the most painful ailment. Low backache is a common complaint in the earlier stages of osteoporosis. In osteoporosis the bones are soft or porous and may be due to a shortage of calcium.

Backache may also be due to constipation, the self-poisoning from absorption of toxic substances from the bowel into the bloodstream. The resulting debilitating state of health robs the back muscles of their normal tone and strength.

Much lower-back troubles can be traced to spinal discs. Small amounts of protruding disc material squeezes out from between the vertebrae and often press on nerves emerging from the spine. Then follows muscle spasm which causes some of the most intense pain.

Abdominal muscles, through lack of exercise, may not give the spine the support it needs from that area. Tough abdominal muscles are a good insurance against disc trouble.

Exercise is then important in relieving and preventing backache. One good exercise is to lie flat on the floor. Put legs in the air and go through a cycling motion. Using a slant-board and cycling while on it is excellent.

Check your posture to be sure it is good. Also look to your shoes. Ill-fitting shoes can have a bad effect on the back.

Diet plays a vital role in developing a strong body which will resist back strain.

Sufficient protein of good quality will build firm tissue which will keep spinal discs properly in place.

B vitamins are of value in treating sciatica, which can result from slipped disc.

To overcome the muscle spasm which causes a great deal of backache, the blood circulation must be improved.

Swamp root, pumpkin seeds, nettle, tansy, uva ursi, buchu and wood betony are the recommended herbs.

Rosinweed root is also said to be good. Place two large tablespoonfuls of the powdered root in one quart of water. Simmer thirty minutes. One cupful four or five times a day is the recommended dose.

Regular, moderate exercise, good posture, good diet, a good back support and a firm mattress are all helpful aids to prevent back trouble.

BAD BREATH

Halitosis has far deeper origins than decaying food remaining in the mouth or decayed teeth.

When the bowels are toxic, the saliva contains indican which causes bad breath.

Bad breath can be caused when fats, stored in the tissues, pass into the bloodstream, circulate to the lungs and then escape in the form of gases.

Also unpleasant gases, formed by offending substances you may have eaten, get into the blood with the assimilation of food. You exhale and you breathe out the offensive odour.

Mouth and tooth infection can cause bad breath, however. Putrefaction of food internally is mostly the direct cause. After toxins and putrefaction are eliminated, foul breath promptly disappears.

Cubeb berries or anise seed may be chewed for offensive breath. Also the gum of cup plant may be chewed to sweeten the breath.

Peppermint tea is said to take away bad breath if taken daily.

BOILS AND CARBUNCLES

Boils and carbuncles are generally caused by infection in a hair follicle. Lowered body resistance against infection may be indicated in the case of boils and carbuncles. Vitamin C will build up resistance to infection.

Poultices made of ground flaxseed, peach tree leaves, catnip leaves or roasted onion and applied hot will draw out the infection. Poultices of yarrow leaves and wheat bran or slippery elm bark (powdered) and lard or plantain leaves boiled and applied hot are also good.

Burdock tea, gentian root, wild cherry bark, nettle, red clover, yellow dock root, sarsaparilla or sassafras are all good alternatives or blood purifiers, and are all good to prevent and keep one free of boils and carbuncles.

Soaking the offending boils or carbuncles in hot epsom salts water when possible is a good aid.

CANCER

Cancer is so widespread that much has been written both to help and also to hinder the finding of a cure for this disease.

Medical science seeks a drug to cure cancer.

A biochemist developed a drug, a chemically synthesized amino acid that is said to have cured leukemia in animals. Why take a synthesized product when a good protein diet will do as much?

Doses of any drug large enough to cure cancer would be strong enough to kill the patient outright.

Marvellous results have been claimed for the grape cure for cancer.

A very good relief for cancer is a tea made of red clover blossoms, either fresh or dried. Drink one quart a day. Violet leaves and flowers should also be added. Other herbs recommended are burdock, yellow dock root, dandelion root, golden seal, slippery elm bark (in cases of stomach cancer especially), comfrey, blue flag, rock rose, and wood betony.

c

For cancer of the breast the following is recommended. Phytolacca, two ounces; Gentian, one ounce; Dandelion Root, one ounce; three pints of water. Simmer to one pint. Make a simple syrup with honey. One teaspoonful after each meal is recommended.

Alkaloids extracted from a periwinkle shrub (Vinca Rosea) is considered one of the most promising anti-cancer agents. Why use an alkaloid? The herb tea is more effective.

I have successfully treated cancer of the skin with the following ointment. Make a very strong tea with red clover blossoms and violet leaves and flowers. The tea is then strained and the liquid is simmered slowly until it is of the consistency of tar. This same ointment was used to remove tumours.

Parsley is rich in potassium and calcium. It has been found that cancer cells cannot multiply in potassium.

Dr. Max Gerson, of Nannet, New York, advocates that cancer cannot develop in normal metabolism. He also said that the liver is the centre of the restoration process in those patients who improve strikingly.

Dr. Harry Goldblatt and his laboratory collaborator at the Institute of Medical Research at Cedar of Lebanon Hospital discovered that normal tissue growing in test tubes becomes cancerous when it is deprived of oxygen. Cancer frequently occurs in scars.

The Drs. Shute, of Canada, in their book *Alpha Tocopherol in Cardiovascular Disease*, point out that vitamin E has been known to reduce the oxygen requirement of muscles by as much as 43%. It is a proven fact that vitamin E will eventually remove scars left by thrombosis.

A resident scientist at Wernse Cancer Research Laboratories at Washington School of Medicine at St. Louis, Missouri, criticized cancer researchers who describe a cure for cancer as being just around the corner, and that a break-through has been discovered. This scientist seemed certain that medical science will never be able to prevent cancer. He also said that people should be aware of cancer-causing substances and be willing to avoid them.

The role of nutrition is an important one in cancer research.

A strong, healthy body will resist the inroads of cancer formation and development.

VIRUS, COUGHS, COLDS AND 'FLU

The common cold causes more actual disability in manhours lost than any other ailment. Although it is the most prevalent ailment in the world, and one of the oldest known to man, it still baffles medical science.

An old remedy consisted of a hot drink, a hot bath, an enema and/or a laxative and rest in bed.

The quicker you get the channels of elimination open, the quicker you will be over a cold.

Sneezing is nature's way of ridding the respiratory tract of the mucous-laden toxina. Never dry up the nasal tract with inhalants. Let nature do her work in a natural sneezy way.

Plenty of alfalfa tea, elderberry and peppermint is a good combination for colds.

A syrup made with a tea of pine needles with lemon juice and honey added, taken hot, is good for a cold. Hot lemonade with mint-flavoured alfalfa tea and honey is also good, if the patient is kept warm in bed.

It is said to be possible to induce a quick recovery from a cold by changing the urine from alkaline to acid by taking two teaspoons of honey and two teaspoons of cider vinegar in a glass of water.

Sore throat has been relieved in one day by chewing the fresh gum from the spruce tree.

A good gargle for sore throat is made with sage, honey and a pinch of cayenne. Another good gargle is made with cider vinegar, salt and a pinch of cayenne.

The following has proved effective in cases of pneumonia. Grease a cloth, spread with ground lobelia herb and heat, and place on chest and on back across the shoulders.

A good combination of herbs for any chest affliction is elecampane, spikenard, rosinweed root and coltsfoot. Steep in boiling water and add enough honey to make a syrup.

Today when one has cold or the 'flu he is said to have a virus.

What is a virus? A virus is supposed to be too small to be seen except with the super-powerful electron microscope and too small to be trapped by the finest filter. It is debatable if they are even alive, yet when one enters a living cell it can do a lot of harm.

Most popular cold remedies contain very dangerous ingredients and are ineffective in fighting a cold. The Lederle Laboratories have gone on record agreeing that antibiotics are ineffective for treating viral respiratory infection.

The British Medical Research Council reported that antihistamines have little or no value in treatment or prevention of colds.

The old-fashioned foot-bath is still good in treating a cold. Keep water as hot as can be borne and add epsom salts. Twenty minutes is not too long to sit with the feet in this bath.

For bronchitis, inhalation of vapours of elderberry blossom tea and camphor is very effective.

Sunflower seeds, along with other herbals, is said to be helpful in bronchitis.

A good remedy for bronchitis is as follows: One cup of red clover blossoms, two level tablespoonfuls of ground flaxseed, one pint boiling water. Mix and steep for one hour. Strain and add honey and the juice of one lemon. Drink hot on going to bed, and cold during the day.

Sage tea is also good for colds and bronchitis.

A good old-fashioned cough syrup is made with hoarhound, slippery elm bark, liquorice root or stick (not the cheap confection) and juice of one lemon. Use honey to make the syrup. Wild cherry bark may also be added.

A hot drink, a hot bath, plenty of juices and liquids and plenty of rest is still the best medication for a cold ever invented.

Diet is an important factor in avoiding winter colds.

You can prevent colds, the 'flu or a virus by taking common-sense care of your health.

CONSTIPATION

Constipation is a thief of good health. Prompt elimination of waste products is vitally important. Delayed elimination may often be the cause of headaches and nervous indigestion. Faulty diet and emotional stress are also causes in a majority of cases.

Artificial means of emptying the bowel disturbs the body chemistry. The body's power of immunity is thus weakened. The use of laxatives depletes the body of potassium, which in turn leads to muscular weakness and often paralysis and myocardial weakness.

Advertising of pharmaceutical companies throws a scare into the public of missed bowel movements and so a fortune is spent yearly on laxatives. It is estimated that Americans spend more than $148,000,000 a year on laxatives.

The use of mineral oil for relief of constipation is widespread. It has been proven that mineral oil interferes with the body's utilization and retention of calcium and phosphorus and interferes with the function of vitamin D.

The adage "an apple a day keeps the doctor away" is certainly true. The use of apple pulp (raw) absorbs poisonous matter in the intestines and carries it downward through the intestines and out of the body. Apple pulp is also good for diarrhoea. Bananas have also been used effectively in diarrhoea, especially in infants.

Adults should drink at least two quarts of water daily. Catnip tea can be used effectively as a drink and also as an enema.

Equal parts of butternut bark, Rocky Mountain grape root, senna leaves and liquorice root makes a good herbal laxative. Cascara Segrada may also be added.

Of course, it is understood that no laxative should ever be given in case of a possible appendicitis.

The best possible way to keep the elimination of waste proceeding naturally and effectively is to eat properly of bulk foods and plenty of vitamins and minerals found in fresh fruits and vegetables.

DIABETES

Diabetes is a condition in which the body cannot utilize all the sugar which enters the bloodstream from digested food. It is a digestive disorder resulting from a deficiency of pancreatic juice. When the secretion of insulin by the pancreas is inhibited, diabetes results. It has been suggested that the liver may be to blame for a breakdown of the pancreas.

The early symptoms are weakness, fatigue, loss in weight in spite of a good appetite, increase of thirst and frequent urination. Carbuncles on the shoulders or scapular region frequently accompanies diabetes.

Doctors are content to control diabetes with insulin rather than attempt to cure it.

A careful diet is better and more effective than inorganic insulin or any of the oral drugs which are harmful. With Orinase, a sulpha drug, there is kidney involvement. Diabinese, even more potent, caused at least forty-three deaths before it was withdrawn from the market.

Dr. Somogyi, in his article in *American Diabetes Association Journal*, stated that by avoiding low blood-sugar, diabetes can be controlled without insulin or drugs.

Insulin is now known to be a zinc molecule. Diabetics may be generally deficient in zinc. Zinc is one of the trace minerals found in herb teas.

Inulin (not insulin) is a carbohydrate which diabetics may eat. It occurs in artichokes, dahlia bulbs and elecampane. Potatoes do not contain inulin.

To assist the pancreas in the manufacture of insulin, the body requires *organic* sulphur. The fruits and vegetables which are rich in sulphur are cabbage, cauliflower, brussels-sprouts, kale, broccoli, collards, onions, leeks, horseradish, watercress, chives, garlic, raspberries, pineapple, currants and apples. These should be eaten raw. Beverage herbs that are rich in sulphur are stinging nettle and fennel seed. It is necessary to balance sulphur herbs with phosphorus herbs. Liquorice root, caraway seed and marigold flowers are some of the phosphorus herbs. Apples contain more phosphorus than any other fruit.

Pine nuts contain no starch and with other nuts make a good source of easily digested protein. All green vegetables may be eaten freely. The early, fresh, succulent vegetables of spring, served raw, are the best remedy for ridding the system of hyperacidity and excess sugar.

Potassium, sodium, calcium, magnesium and iron are the recommended minerals. Beverage herbs containing these minerals are black walnut leaves, camomile flowers, eyebright, stinging nettle, comfrey, fennel seeds and strawberry leaves. Dandelion greens in early spring are also good.

There have been cases where, after drinking a tea of huckleberry leaves for several months instead of water, there was no trace of sugar in the urine. The same effect was obtained after drinking a tea of crawlgrass for several months.

Roots of the "devil's club", a prickly shrub, was used by American Indians for diabetes.

A tea made of soy bean pods, oat straw and wild carrot tops has also proven effective. Soy bean pod tea seems to successfully lower the sugar level of the blood.

A vitamin C deficiency may be the underlying cause of diabetes. Vitamin B helps to cut down on insulin intake. Lemon juice, unsweetened and diluted, oxidizes excess blood sugar.

The brain depends upon the moment to moment blood-sugar level for its functioning. This may be attributed to the blackouts that occur in diabetes.

Diabetes may return if you go on a cake and candy binge! Persevere in an intelligent diet including beverage herbs if you wish to be free from diabetes.

EARS THAT HEAR

Impairment of hearing ranks fourth among the top handicapping illnesses.

Many who become hard of hearing, especially after middle-age, do not need a hearing aid. Often wax collects in the ear canals, and, when removed by a doctor, hearing is often restored in minutes. It is best to let a doctor remove the wax for two reasons. First, the ear is a delicate organ and can be easily injured. Secondly, as in one case, the wax hardened on the eardrum. If not removed carefully in such a case, inflammation of the brain could follow.

If deafness is not caused by wax, there is still hope for the hard of hearing. In 1949 a world famous ear specialist connected with a large New York hospital held the theory that deafness is caused by an excess of pyruvic acid in the bloodstream. To help correct this condition, which is caused by faulty carbohydrate metabolism, he advocated the use of B-amino complex.

EYES THAT SEE

The one part of the body which reacts more readily to conditions of poor health is the eyes. Regardless of what organ may be diseased, the signs first appear in the eyes.

As long ago as 400 B.C., Hippocrates fed his patients the livers of birds to cure blindness. In the last forty years, science has proved why this cure worked.

A normal, wholesome diet will help to prevent and even cure such eye conditions as poor vision, abnormal sensitivity to glare and bright lights and other eye conditions.

Continued errors in food intake rob your eyes of precious elements so necessary to good eye health. Better food habits could free everyone of eye disorders and eye glasses could be outmoded.

The public should be warned about optic nerve degeneration and even complete blindness due to side-effects of drugs. People are led to believe that drugs are the only answer to curing disease. Side-effects of drugs are more harmful than the original illness. Thiouracil, commonly used for depression of an overactive thyroid, has caused paralysis of the muscles of the eyes and of the eyelids, causing them to droop. It has also interfered with the focusing power of the eye. Prolonged use of acetophenetidin, a common ingredient in aspirin, also affects the eyes. Atropine, used in eye examination and also for motion sickness, interferes with the eyes' accommodation to light and darkness. Potassium iodide can cause degeneration of the retina. The prolonged use of chloramphenicol results in the degeneration of the optic nerve and also interferes with the assimilation and synthesis of the B vitamins.

Contact lenses have been linked to blindness. According to Dr. William Stone, Director of the Ophthalmic Plastic Research Laboratories at the Massachusetts Eye and Ear Infirmary of Boston, methacrylic acid, used in the manufacture of the plastic which is used in making contact lenses, is sometimes retained in the plastic after it is hardened. Tears caused by irritation can draw the acid from the lenses and, depending upon the amount of acid present, can cause serious damage to the eyes.

Boric acid, often used in treating the eyes has caused death in some instances (*JAMA*, December 28, 1963).

Prolonged deficiency of certain food factors lead to cataract. A deficiency of riboflavin and calcium has been found to produce cataract. About one-fifth of all cases of slight loss of sight are caused by cataract.

Glaucoma is a hardening of the arteries of the eyeball. About 2½% of all people over 40 contract glaucoma. It is extremely painful, especially at the onset.

There is convincing evidence that cortisone-like drugs can cause hardening of the eyeball.

The purity of the bloodstream is of special importance in curing glaucoma. Toxic waste must be eliminated. This elimination is best begun by fasting, followed with fruit and vegetable juice therapy. Then a balanced diet with special emphasis on vitamin A and riboflavin has been recommended. Such a diet is also important in treating cataract.

Spinal manipulation has also been indicated.

Sunflower seeds seem to be a specific for good vision. Sunflower seeds are rich in the B vitamins. The oil in the seeds is very rich in vitamins A and D. The seeds are also rich in calcium, phosphorus and iron, all of which are known to be valuable to good eye health.

There are also herbs which, when taken as a tea, will improve eye health.

In an Old English herbal, horehound tea and wine and honey is said to "clear the eyesight".

Juniper berries are said to fortify the sight by strengthening the optic nerve.

Old herbalists claimed that elecampane "clears, strengthens and quickens the sight of the eyes wonderfully".

Another herbalist claimed that eyebright "hath restored sight to them that have been blind a long time before".

Rosemary is said to "clear dim sight".

A report by a famous Swedish botanist, Peter Kalm, tells how a Mohawk Medicine Man restored the sight of an Indian boy after all other known methods and remedies of the time were tried and failed. The fumes or vapour from a decoction of witch hazel bark was passed through a funnel that was held near the eye. The boy had been blind for six months.

A quaint old rhyme goes like this:

> Noble is Rue! It makes the sight of the eyes
> both sharp and clear;
> With the help of Rue, oh! blear-eyed man!
> Thou shalt see far and near.

Culpeper made the claim that "Eyebright made into a powder and then into an electuary (a syrup) with honey, hath a powerful effect and help to restore the sight decayed by age".

Pliny said in his writings that the Pythagoreans believed that the absence of blindness and eye trouble in general was attributed to the daily consumption of honey.

A good drink that will keep the sparkle in your eyes is made as follows: Place one cup of raw carrot juice, one level teaspoonful of rosehips powder, one egg yolk, a little honey, ground sunflower seeds and sesame seeds, one teaspoonful of brewer's yeast, one-quarter cup of eyebright tea, and a pinch of kelp in the blender, and blend well. It is delicious and an eye-brightner.

A good eyewash may be made by mixing fennel seed, camomile flowers and eyebright. Steep in boiling water and strain through a cloth to remove all residue. Apply with an eye-cup.

For pink eye, scrape Irish potato and apply to eyes. Also sassafrass pith made into a tea and applied with an eyedropper. All teas dropped into the eyes must be strained through a clean cloth to remove any sediment.

One of the worst things that can happen to you is blindness. Take the very best care of you eyes while you can still see. They come only two to a customer.

EPILEPSY

Epilepsy is more prevalent than might be thought. One out of every one hundred persons suffers from epilepsy.

More than fifty years ago the first epilepsy colony was established in the State of New York. It was advocated there that hard muscular work is a good remedy for epilepsy. The superintendent of the colony announced that the patients worked off the convulsions at the end of a hoe handle by vigorous field work.

It has been proven that active muscular work is almost a panacea in cases of epilepsy in which the brain has not been damaged.

Epilepsy is not incurable, as once thought.

Diet is very important in epilepsy therapy. The following suggestions should be carried out. First, cut down on all liquids. Secondly, cut down on all starch foods. Thirdly, increase fats (unsaturated). Fourthly, no milk, no pork, fried or refined foods should be eaten. And lastly, no ice cream, canned fruit or rich desserts should be allowed.

Spinal alignment, particularly in the upper cervical area, has been proven effective.

In epilepsy therapy avoid excitement, overeating, improper rest, poor elimination, intoxicants and refined food products.

Glutamic acid is said to be effective. Glutamic acid is one of the essential amino acids. It is found in eggs, meat, cheese, beans and fish. Glutamic acid should never be taken alone in its isolated state.

Since epilepsy affects the nervous system, the calmative tea, skuppcap, nerve root, valerian, catnip and peppermint is good.

Blue vervain may be added to the foregoing formula or taken alone, since it has been used effectively in epilepsy therapy as well as for nervous conditions.

Ephedrin is also used in the treatment of epilepsy. Ephedrin is extracted from MaHuang. Ephedrin is also found in Mormon Valley herb, or Herb of the Sun, as it is also called.

Eyebright has also been found effective. Take four fluid ounces of the tea on an empty stomach and at bed time.

The following single herbs have also been found effective: Elder flowers, black cohosh, blue cohosh and hyssop, which is excellent.

ERUPTIVE DISEASES

Chicken pox: Senna, one ounce; elder flowers, one ounce; pleurisy root, one ounce; yarrow, one ounce; and ginger, quarter ounce.

Measles and scarlet fever: Saffron.

Scarlet fever: Equal parts of pleurisy root, vervain, ground ivy, red sage and centaury.

Smallpox: Wood sage, pitcher plant, valerian, saffron, peppermint, each one ounce; marigold flowers, one-half ounce.

As a preventive against smallpox, place one ounce each of pitcher plant and ground ivy in two pints of boiling water. Simmer down to one pint. Take one tablespoonful every six hours. One-half teaspoonful cream of tartar in a glass of water is also good as a preventive of smallpox and taken after having the disease.

FEVERS

When the body is filled with waste matter, fever is nature's way of burning up the impurities. It acts as a germ killer and enables the body to rid itself of any ailment.

In Central America and Mexico a plant grows which is known as fever flowers. The natives call it "Jamaica". It is used in that part of the country to allay fevers. The flower petals make a delightful, thirst-satisfying drink very similar to lemonade.

Pennyroyal is fine to break up ague and chills.

One-half teaspoonful of cream of tartar is also good in fevers.

Cascara, Orgeon grape root and princess pine have relieved cases of malaria.

A tea made of elderberry blossoms will help to relieve a fever. Yarrow tea is said to relieve a fever in twenty-four hours if taken one teaspoonful every thirty minutes.

Other fever herbs are catnip, shepherd's purse, sumach berries, tansy, thyme, valerian, wahoo bark, wild cherry bark, borage, apple tree bark, camomile, calamus, nettle, parsley, peppermint, sarsaparilla, bonset and sage.

Sponge a fever patient with common baking soda water.

If no milk is given and fruit and vegetable juices (raw) are given (no solid food), a fever can be reduced in a few hours.

HEADACHE

Headache is a very common ailment. In most cases, headaches are symptoms of some disorder in the body.

Headaches may be caused by toxaemia, excitement, fatigue, biliousness, indigestion, constipation, high blood pressure, eye strain, a liver disorder or a case of the nerves. Women often suffer a form of frontal headache which may be caused by a genital disorder.

Some doctors consider tension headache and migraine as one and the same.

Migraine headache may be caused by a low blood-sugar level.

Headache is a danger signal. When a certain organ of the body is not functioning normally, nature gives a warning.

Therefore it is very unwise to resort to aspirin or other pain-killing drugs to alleviate pain. You may dull the pain, but the source of trouble is still there and eventually may result in greater disturbances.

Take a cupful of strong, hot peppermint tea. Lie down and relax a while. Your headache will soon be gone. Try this in place of aspirin.

A hot foot bath with a cold towel around the head may ease the suffering.

Wring out a cloth in a hot solution of hop tea and diluted cider vinegar and apply to the head.

For migraine or other headaches, put equal parts of vinegar and water in a small pan and allow to boil slowly. When vapours begin to rise, hold the head over it and inhale. This is said to stop the headache in a half hour.

Catnip, nerve root, blue scullcap, valerian and peppermint are a good herb combination to take for headache.

Migraine responds to vitamin therapy, especially the B vitamins.

Experiments have proved that a good protein breakfast will almost without exception completely relieve headache.

It has also been found that migraine sufferers may be allergic to sodium propionate, which is widely used as a preservative in many foods, including bread and also in tobacco.

It has also been suggested that chocolate may trigger migraine.

A new drug, Methyseridge, is claimed to cure migraine. However, there have been cases where the patient developed swelling of the ankles, legs and thighs, cramp in the calves, a rapid increase in weight, severe indigestion and rapid falling out of the hair.

For any headache, the barbiturates are dangerous. They tend to increase the intracellular pressure on the brain cells.

From the very first you experience headache, stop eating. Drink plenty of pure water or lemon water. Clean out the bowels with a catnip enema. Have the spine checked. Watch your diet and get plenty of rest. Neck-stretching has also been advocated.

If you try to carry the world on your shoulders, you will soon experience head pain.

THE AILING HEART

Without the proper functioning of the heart, there would be no life.

Heart disease kills more people than any other disease. Deaths from heart disease have increased 50% in the last ten years.

Knowing how to care for your heart is all-important.

Our forefathers did hard physical labour. They ate large quantities of fresh wholegrains such as wheat, corn, rye and millet which contain the raw, unrefined oils which are known to protect the heart and blood vessels. Today, fresh wholegrain has almost entirely disappeared from most diets.

There is much discussion today on the use of vitamin E in the treatment of coronary thrombosis since the medical team of Drs. Wilfred E Shute and Evan Shute, of Canada, developed the use of vitamin E in the treatment of heart ailments.

In their book, *Your Heart and You*, is much information on the use of vitamin E. It is one of the best sources of information on cardiac ailments and is reliable.

Vitamin E is a complex of several factors. Alpha tocopherol is the factor best to use in the treatment of heart disease. Alpha tocopherol opens up a whole new avenue of hope to heart sufferers.

Modern advertising has made the public cholesterol conscious. Cholesterol is a fatty substance which builds up and clogs the arteries, making it harder for the heart to function, putting a severe strain upon the heart. Research has found that unrefined vegetable oils depress or neutralize the cholesterol in the blood.

Mer/29 or Triparanol is a drug intended for reducing blood cholesterol. The purpose of this drug is to lower body cholesterol by inhibiting its being produced by the body. No interference should ever be made with the body's own ability to produce cholesterol or any other secretion.

Excessive straining during a bowel movement may cause a series of circulatory changes that might end with the dislodging of a thrombus.

Underfunctioning of the adrenal and thyroid glands has been found in many cardiac patients.

Perhaps the greatest cause of heart disease is wrong diet.

The heart is a tough muscle. However, if deficiencies are continued over a long period of time, the heart suffers.

A subnormal level of vitamin C has been found in most cardiac patients.

It has also been found that Pangamic acid (B-15) helps the heart to function properly. B-15 has been discovered in certain foods which are also sources of the B complex, especially in brewer's yeast and seeds.

Sudden noise or excitement can cause palpitation of the heart. This is an annoyance rather than a disease. Persons of calm temperaments who exercise control over their emotions are rarely troubled with palpitation. Palpitation may also be caused by gas and fermentation in the stomach. Tansy tea is a specific for palpitation of the heart.

According to Dr. Paul Dudley White, of Boston, the famous heart specialist, indigestion can lead to a wrong diagnosis of coronary heart disease. Cardiospasm is the commonest condition with which coronary heart disease may be confused. The cardiospasm pain tends to be briefer and recurrent, comes on in time of rest and is often dispelled by walking or the belching of gas.

There are herbs that can help to strengthen the heart. A good combination is golden seal, scullcap and a pinch of cayenne. Some have used wild cherry bark to strengthen the heart. However, a very small amount of the wild cherry should be used.

Another good combination is golden seal, scullcap, nerve root, valerian, camomile and a pinch of cayenne.

There are different types of heart disease. Most heart trouble can be overcome. Reasonable care of this organ can give you every chance of living a normal life span. However, because of its serious nature, it is best to see your doctor.

HAEMORRHOIDS

Haemorrhoids or piles, as they are commonly known, are enlarged veins of the rectum caused by an obstruction in the return circulation. Constipation is a common cause of haemorrhoids. Lubricants, hot and cold sitz baths and regulating the bowels may be of help.

Simmer garlic powder and cocoa butter. Make into suppositories. Insert one after each bowel movement and at bedtime. Powdered garlic mixed with lanolin is also good. Simmer elder bark in grease. Apply to afflicted part after each bowel movement. Mullein leaves, balm of gilead buds, peach tree leaves or cheese plant may be used in this way.

HICCOUGHS

Sipping water slowly is an old remedy for hiccoughs. Tea made of the dill plant given in teaspoon doses is also said to be good. Often a few mint leaves well chewed will stop hiccoughs. Caraway tea is also said to be beneficial. Pineapple juice is also helpful. Cases of hiccoughs have been helped with watermelon seeds (tea) after all other remedies failed.

Pressure for two or three minutes on each side of the neck about one inch below the ears has been found helpful.

Hiccoughs is a spasmodic contraction of the diaphragm caused by gas in the stomach. Calamus and peppermint are excellent to remove gas from the stomach.

HIGH BLOOD PRESSURE

High blood pressure is the body's danger signal that there is trouble ahead.

What causes high blood pressure or hypertension, as it is called professionally, is still a medical mystery.

There are many theories advocated. Experiments point to an insufficient blood supply to the kidneys. Overweight is also said to be a cause of high blood pressure. It is also thought to be a loss of harmony within the circulatory system. The heart and blood vessels are so harmonized that they will work normally if they are not abused.

Wrong eating and drinking habits, accompanied by poor

D

elimination, are chief causes of high blood pressure. It is also caused by worry, fretting, anxiety and anger.

One thing is certain. There is some connection between high blood pressure and the tension of modern living. Working under constant strain and emotion-charged problems can trigger blood pressure levels.

Low blood pressure rarely if ever causes trouble unless it is extremely low. The number of people in whom low blood pressure is a serious danger is comparatively small.

If the blood pressure remains consistently high for a long period of time, it can result in serious damage to the heart.

Dangerously high blood pressure may be lowered to safer levels when an overweight person reduces his weight.

Restriction of salt should be in high blood pressure therapy.

Only four days on a protein supplement (40 grams daily) has lowered blood pressure.

Learning to relax will prevent high blood pressure and reduce it when necessary.

The arteries are so well constructed that they should last an individual one hundred years. They will renew themselves if the blood is kept pure, and they will remain soft and pliable. When the walls of the blood vessels toughen, blood pressure soars.

Three hundred and thirty three mgs of vitamin C, three times a day, has proved effective in lowering blood pressure.

Rest is imperative. A warm bath at night and plenty of sleep in a well-ventilated room will do much to lower blood pressure. An afternoon nap can reduce blood pressure 15 to 30 points and calm jittery nerves.

Garlic has been proven clinically to lower blood pressure. Mistletoe has been found excellent for dizziness caused by high blood pressure. Cayenne and watermelon seeds have also been proved to be effective.

Black cohosh, blue cohosh, valerian, scullcap, golden seal and vervain are recommended herbs for high blood pressure problems. The calmative tea, scullcap, nerve root, valerian, catnip and peppermint will work wonders to lower blood-pressure levels.

KIDNEY AND BLADDER DISORDERS

The main work of excretion is performed by the kidneys. The kidneys are blood purifiers.

When the urine analysis shows albumin, it is evidence that the kidneys are involved.

Kidneys may be slowed up by protein-rich and uric-acid forming foods, by irritating acids caused by colds and by weakness and fatigue. Worry, overwork, wrong food and drink. cold and exposure put a strain upon the kidneys.

To clear up sluggish kidneys drink herb teas, eliminate meat and other proteins for a time and live on a simple diet. Plenty of fruit and vegetable juices are recommended.

Salt and other condiments put special strain on the kidneys. Also constant use of alcohol, drugs and chemical irritants affect the kidneys.

Plenty of fresh air and sunshine, bathing, massage and mild exercise help the kidneys in their function. There will be less strain on the kidneys when the skin and lungs are in condition to function properly.

Since the kidneys and bladder are correlated in their function of excretion, the same medication is suitable for both.

The following herbs are recommended in kidney and bladder disorders. Swamp lily root, marshmallow root, cheese plant, buchu leaves, corn silk, juniper berries and wahoo bark. A tea of caraway seeds is recommended for irritation of the bladder.

The residents of the Cape Cod area drink cranberry juice for relief from kidney and bladder infection. Cranberries contain quinic acid, which is converted into hitturic acid, which in turn is effective as a deterrent to the formation of kidney stones.

In the case of dropsy, horsetail and wahoo bark are recommended. The following formula is also effective in treating dropsy: Juniper berries, stinging nettle, yarrow, rosemary and horsetail grass.

Waste substances resulting from the function of other organs include ammonia, uric acid, creatin and sulphuric acid. If these substances are not excreted properly and promptly, they become potent enough to cause physical impairment. Urinary disorders may develop into such ailments as nephritis or Bright's Disease and nephrosis.

GALL BLADDER

The chief function of the gall bladder is the collection and storage and concentration of bile which comes from the liver.

Removal of the gall bladder is a common practice. You can get along without a gall bladder, but digestion will never be the same. Bile is used to emulsify fats and oils. The body cannot use fats unless they are emulsified. When the gall bladder is removed, much of the fats and oils are lost, having no food value.

The diet is a matter of first importance in gall bladder trouble.

A famous Dutch physician found that the gall bladder of oxen at the end of winter were filled with calculi (stones), but fresh spring pasturage dissipated these stones. Fresh vegetables and vegetable juices are the best remedy for dissolving these stones.

Foods with a fair content of sulphur will also correct this condition. Radishes are especially recommended.

Fresh fruit juices diluted with water, manipulated to the spinal areas which affect the nerve controls of the gall bladder, principally the neck and the fifth and ninth dorsal vertebrae, are all good in nature's way of curing gall stones.

Herbs suggested for gall-bladder trouble are gobernadora and vervain.

Treatment with the sulphas, antibiotics and bladder sedation has not proved satisfactory. Herb teas and proper diet is the best answer to gall-bladder trouble.

The best cure is always prevention. A high state of vitality and good health must be maintained to avoid gall-bladder disorder.

LIVER DISORDERS

The liver is the largest and one of the most important organs of the body. It serves as a regulator of the body. The bile which it produces is to the intestines what the gastric juice is to the stomach. The work of the liver is important to the entire body.

The relation of the kidneys and liver is important in the elimination of waste.

The liver is the control centre of the entire system, of all body chemistry.

One of the big jobs of the liver is to clean out of the blood such substances as would harm us physically. If the liver is sluggish, it does not do its job of filtering waste quickly enough or completely enough.

Among other essential liver functions is the maintenance of sex hormone balance. The liver's part in this is so sensitive that liver ailments may cause feminizing manifestations in men, and women whose livers are sluggish may experience menstrual difficulties and pain.

Indigestion is connected with liver complaints, for the liver controls the assimilation of food.

Hepatitis is a very common ailment today. Hepatitis is a professional term meaning infection of the liver. It is also called jaundice.

Diet is tremendously important in restoring the liver to healthful functioning. All sugars, alcohol, fried foods and condiments should be avoided.

All the components of the B complex are suggested for regenerating a diseased liver. Also from 300–600 mgs of organic vitamin C and not less than 750 mgs of calcium.

Sulphur foods are valuable for secretion of bile and for overcoming enlarged liver since it promotes the flow of bile.

Vitamin E is also a vital factor in the health and normalcy of the liver.

Plenty of the B complex is recommended to keep the liver working properly. B-12 is also extremely important to aid the liver in its functioning.

It has been found that Epsom salts will stir a sluggish liver.

The following combination of herbs is very helpful in restoring the liver to proper functioning. Rocky Mountain grape root, dandelion root, sarsaparilla, may apple root and golden seal.

Mandrake root, black soot, sacred bark, colic root and blue vervain are recommended herbs.

The following combination of herbs is also good. One ounce dandelion root, one-half ounce each of mandrake, sarsaparilla, blackberry root and buchu, one and one-half ounces of gentian and one handful of hops. Three cups of this tea should be taken daily.

Grate winter radishes, sprinkle with salt and let stand three hours. One teaspoonful every three hours is the recommended amount to take.

The laxative effect of certain herbs is of great importance since most liver and gall bladder disorders are accompanied by constipation. Raw juice of dandelion leaves, stinging nettle, watercress and cabbage is excellent in treating the liver.

In the treatment of the liver, chemicals are only an additional burden to the already damaged organ.

In spite of the liver's special self-preservation ability, liver disease was listed in 1962 as one of the top ten causes of death between the ages of 45 and 64.

A highly nutritious diet with plenty of bed-rest is advocated by most physicians in the treatment of hepatitis.

Keep your liver in good condition by not overeating, choosing a proper, wholesome diet, drink herb teas, breathe deeply and exercise freely.

MULTIPLE SCLEROSIS

Just what is the cause of multiple sclerosis has not been fully ascertained. Eventually it may be proved to be a disease of malnutrition and best treated nutritionally.

Non-civilized races do not have this disease. However, when they come in contact with the diet of civilization they begin to contract multiple sclerosis.

In multiple sclerosis patients there is an abnormal blood–sugar level and a calcium deficiency. Excessive amounts of carbohydrates cause skyrocketing rises and falls in blood–sugar.

Improvement in multiple sclerosis patients has been obtained with the B vitamins. B vitamins are necessary for proper functioning of the carbohydrate metabolism.

Multiple sclerosis is thought to be a disorder of fat metabolism. A diet rich in fats, especially animal fats, may be one of the factors which brings on this disease.

Billions of favourable bacteria are in the normal intestine. Antibiotics kill all the intestinal flora as well as pyridoxin, which in turn causes a niacin deficiency. Without pyridoxin, niacin becomes a poison. Also, tryptophan, one of the essential aminos, cannot be used properly. This condition in the intestines can also act on the mylin, the fatty protein sheath covering the nerves. When no pyridoxin is present, the myelin breaks down and nerves are damaged. Myelin damage is the basic symptom of multiple sclerosis. Since the myelin sheath is a protein substance, a sufficient supply of good protein in the diet would be valuable in maintaining the proper strength and thickness of this nerve covering. Chemical drugs also destroy these favourable bacteria in the intestines.

A suggested diet in multiple sclerosis consists of plenty of good protein, no white sugar or carbohydrates, plenty of calcium, vitamin B complex (brewer's yeast), desiccated liver kelp, safflower oil and rosehips.

A good combination of nerve herbs should be of special help in multiple sclerosis.

The general health is a major factor in reducing the number of cases of this dreaded disease.

MUSCULAR DYSTROPHY

Muscular dystrophy now affects some 200,000 people or one person in 925.

It is plain to research scientists that nutrition is the main factor in muscular dystrophy. Dys means, literally, imperfect or faulty nutrition.

A depression of the potassium content of the body has been noted in most patients with muscular dystrophy.

Herbs containing potassium are walnut leaves, mistletoe, camomile, calamus, plantain leaves, eyebright, summer savoury, carrot leaves, fennel seed, comfrey, dandelion and stinging nettle.

The absence of choline can cause progressive muscular dystrophy in rabbits.

Vitamin E is also considered in the cause of this disease. When massive doses of vitamin E are given in research experiments, the muscles returned to normal.

Wheat germ oil has been used with good effect in treating muscular dystrophy. In a reported treatment of twenty-five muscular dystrophy patients with wheat germ oil, vitamin B and vitamin C, all improved and one recovered completely.

Large doses of inositol and vitamin E together have helped in the treating of muscular dystrophy.

NERVOUSNESS

We are living in a nervous age. Stress, tension, worry and poor diet all contribute to a case of the nerves.

Good elimination is most essential in nervous conditions. Hot then cold fomentations to the spine are beneficial in nervous ailments, followed by gentle back massage. Also hot packs held to the back of the neck help to relax.

The nervous system is strengthened most by foods which give an alkaline reaction, foods which are rich in potassium, sodium, calcium, magnesium, iron and phosphorus. Herb teas containing these minerals are just as helpful.

The best herb formula I have found for nervousness is as follows: Nerve root, skullcap, valerian, peppermint and catnip.

For St. Vitus Dance, the following has proved helpful: A combination of equal parts of skullcap and lady's slipper. Another combination of herbs which are said to be effective in treating St. Vitus Dance is equal parts of skullcap, mistletoe, St. John's wort, valerian, gentian and a very small part of lobelia.

For NERVOUS HEADACHE, pour one quart of boiling water on one-half ounce each of camomile and peppermint. Drink freely.

A good NERVINE is made with skullcap, motherwort, black

cohosh, valerian and wood betony. Also, equal parts of scullcap, valerian, mistletoe, hops and powdered liquorice make a good nervine.

A tea made of garden sage is good for nerve exhaustion. Garlic is also said to be a good nerve tonic. Camomile, celery seeds and tops, and hops are also good taken in combination or as single herbs.

The brain, heart, stomach, liver, pancreas, spleen and every other vital organ, every muscle and every cell is governed by the nerves. The individual with a well-balanced nervous system, a pure bloodstream and an alert mind feels on top of the world.

To ensure a stong nervous system, sleep more, exercise more, eat a wholesome diet, worry less and live at a slower tempo. Take time to laugh. It is a safety valve.

NEURALGIA

B-12 injection is excellent for relief in neuralgia. Hot catnip tea is also good.

NEURITIS

Lack of vitamin B is evidenced in neuritis. Rocky Mountain grape root is said to be effective in treating neuritis.

PAIN

Pain is not a disease. It is merely a symptom. It means that a nerve has been irritated.

The dangerous drug aspirin is probably the worst remedy ever foisted upon the public.

Aspirin is a trade name. It is used to describe a substance known as acetylsalicylic acid, a coal-tar product. It is doubly dangerous because, in suppressing symptoms, it gives one a false sense that everything is all right.

Habitual use of over-the-counter medication to relieve pain constitutes a serious threat to health.

The long continued use of phenacetin, one of the ingredients in some pain pills, accounts for a number of anaemia and kidney diseases. The charges against phenacetin are enought to disqualify any product containing it as a safe medication.

It has been reported that salicylates interfere with the production of hormones by the thyroid gland.

Two or three aspirins cause an increased flow of blood from the stomach lining. One professor of a graduate school of medicine pointed out that aspirin causes internal bleeding and may lead to ulcers and anaemia.

Allergic reaction to aspirin can be violent in persons afflicted with asthma.

Sales of aspirin and aspirin-containing compounds in the U.S.A. totalled more than $282,000,000 during 1960. Advertising by aspirin manufacturers has proved a profitable business.

Instead of aspirin and the host of pain relievers on the market, wisdom points to herbs to relieve pain.

A combination of five plants for fast pain relief are valerian, scullcap, passion flower, balm of gilead buds, willow bark, black cohosh, hops and lady slipper with brewer's yeast and B-12 added to the diet.

Althea or marshmallow root is pain soothing.

A burdock leaf poultice will allay inflammation and ease pain. Wilt the leaf and apply to the affected part.

For the pain of sinus infection, neuralgia and arthritis, one teaspoon apple cider vinegar in a glass of water four times a day for two weeks has been suggested. Pain is associated with alkaline urine reaction. Cider vinegar changes the urine to an acid reaction.

Pain is greatly exaggerated when there is a lack of phosphorus and potassium.

The phosphorus and potassium herbs are walnut leaves, camomile flowers, calamus, plantain leaves, coltsfoot, eyebright, summer savoury, stinging nettle, borage, dandelion leaves, comfrey, fennel seed, yarrow, mullein, carrot leaves, caraway seed, marigold flowers, and liquorice root.

Besides relieving pain, these herbs supply valuable minerals and are harmless.

POLIO

Really healthy children do not get polio. Dr. Benjamin Sandler was of that opinion. He stopped a North Carolina polio epidemic by going to the newspapers and television with a special diet. Worried parents followed his diet faithfully. The polio cases dropped almost magically.

Those who are interested may read for themselves Dr. Sandler's book, *Diet Prevents Polio*, published by the Lee Foundation for Nutritional Research, 2023 W. Wisconsin Avenue, Milwaukee, Wisconsin.

Four cases of paralytic polio were reported in Canada after they had received the oral type polio vaccine.

A two-year-old California boy was stricken with paralysis in his legs fifteen days after taking Type III Sabin oral polio vaccine.

Investigation of a Nebraska polio outbreak showed that nine persons developed an illness comparable with acute polio between seven to twenty-two days after taking Type III oral vaccine.

An article in a German medical journal reviewed 150 cases of muscle paralysis following vaccination with Type I.

In several English medical journals it was shown that polio cases were due to inocculation for diphtheria and whooping cough.

A New York City doctor blamed the upsurge of polio cases to vitamin A deficiency.

Vitamin B therapy has been found effective in polio and sleeping sickness.

There is also a polio risk after tonsillectomies.

Begin treatment for polio with hot, moist flannels applied to painful, contracted muscles. When the muscles become relaxed, skilful manipulation of the limb should be given by one who knows the human muscular system. When the patient is able, he should be encouraged to move the limb himself until he can do it without help.

After pressing a nerve in the knee, the feet and arms are said to come back to place.

When the patient is able to, have him stretch until every part of the spine is involved.

Hot and cold applications to the spine have also proved effective.

The following herbs are recommended in polio cases: Valerian, dandelion root, scullcap, golden seal, black cohosh, catnip, red clover blossoms and yellow dock. Select one or several and mix in equal parts. An excellent combination is made as follows: Equal parts of valerian, catnip, scullcap and sweet flag root. These herbs are harmless.

PROSTATE TROUBLE

The prostate is a male sex gland. After middle-age it is a potential troublemaker. After middle-age, more than 60% of all men experience prostate trouble. Much of this distress can be overcome.

There are men who have defeated surgery by adopting better nutritional habits. The fat-soluble vitamins seem to be associated with the health of the prostate.

Modern medical science has not been able to find a successful method of therapy other than surgery.

A hot sitz bath (105 to 115 degrees), in which the lower part of the body is soaked for twenty minutes to an hour, has a soothing effect and may reduce the swelling.

In 1958, Dr. W. Devrient, of Berlin, Germany, cured his patients of prostate trouble by having them eat pumpkin seeds.

There is evidence of a decrease in zinc content in glands containing malignant tissue. Pumpkin seeds are specific for a healthy prostate since they have a high zinc content. Other zinc-rich foods are brewer's yeast, onions, rice bran, eggs, nuts, seeds, molasses, peas, beans, wheat germs, wheat bran, oysters and beef liver.

Lecithin has been suggested by twenty-one researchers as curative of enlarged prostate gland. Seeds of all kinds are rich in lecithin.

Parsley gives relief in prostate pressure.

One-half teaspoon powered slippery elm bark mixed with warm water to make a lumpless paste, with one-half glass of warm water, and drunk morning and evening, has been effective in severe agonizing cases of prostate trouble.

Peach tree leaves are said to be good in cases of prostate trouble. Cornsilk, golden seal, buchu and garlic are also recommended. Blue flag has special action on the prostate gland.

Herb teas are more effective when used in conjunction with a good wholesome diet.

SALVES AND LINIMENTS

LINIMENT
Vinegar (apple cider), 1 pint
Cayenne, 1 teaspoonful
Hops
Black cohosh
Lobelia
Camphorated oil
Peppermint oil

SALVE (1)
Red clover blossoms
"Life everlasting"
Yarrow
Elderberry blossoms
Golden seal
Wheat germ oil
Arnica flowers
Balm of Gilead buds

SALVE (2)
Elderberry blossoms
Yarrow
Red clover blossoms
Golden seal
Balm of Gilead buds

GRANDPA'S LINIMENT
Ague ammonia 1 oz.
Tincture arnica, ½ oz.
Gum camphor, ½ oz.
Oil turpentine, ¼ oz.
Olive oil, ¼ oz.
Oil peppermint, ¼ oz.
Alcohol, ¼ pint

This salve (2) was used on third-degree burns and left no scar.

Other good ointments to be used on burns are as follows:
Oil of pennyroyal and raw linseed oil.
Elderberry blossoms, yarrow and red clover blossoms simmered in vegetable oil.

Chestnut leaves steeped and applied to burns.
Chopped leaves of aloes (aloe vera) applied to burns.
Tannic acid is an old remedy for burns.
Aloes are good for X-ray burns.

Cod liver oil has healing properties. It kills harmful organisms. The application of cod liver oil dressings to infected wounds in fifty-three patients was very effective in combating infection. Researchers found that the growth of streptococci is stopped within one hour and the growth of staphylococci is stopped at the end of six hours when cod liver oil is used.

Wonderful results are reported in treating wounds with honey. Dip gauze in honey and apply. Change dressing daily.

To draw out pus, add all the Epsom salts to any good salve that it will hold and still remain spreadable.

Salve made from comfrey root will heal wounds and is said to cause broken bones and fractures to knit.

A Veratrain ointment is said to remove bullets without surgery. Webster's dictionary lists Veratrain as being an extract from the sabadilla seeds. American Hellebore is also known as Veratrum Veride. Someone might like to investigate further.

MOTION SICKNESS

If the liver functions normally, attacks of motion sickness may be prevented.

Do not begin an air trip or voyage on an empty stomach. A bowl of warm soup, especially if the weather is cold or cheerless, may keep you from the rail. Shun any food on the trip which you know will cause gas.

Do not get into a dither for some days before starting.

Keep the bowels open, It is advocated that one take a good cathartic before starting on a trip.

Take a quarter teaspoonful cayenne pepper in a bowl of hot soup. All sickness, nausea and squeamishness will disappear.

Preludin, the anti-seasickness drug, has been banned from

use in the Scandinavian countries. Atropine is also a dangerous drug and should not be used in cases of motion sickness.

SHINGLES

No case of shingles is without emotional upset or emotional strain.

In treating shingles, give an enema every day, whether the bowels move or not. Clean out the system fast. Complete abstinence of all white sugar, white flour and fried foods is of the utmost importance.

A good supplement of 750–1500 mgs of calcium, 300 mgs vitamin C and the whole B complex is recommended.

SINUSITIS

An unbearable pain in the head and congestion in the sinus region are characteristic of sinus trouble.

The only real relief can be found in a non-mucous-forming diet. Starches should be the first food to be eliminated from the daily diet.

Acidosis is always present in sinus infection. Milk, meat, fish, cheese, and cereals are acid-forming. These foods must be balanced with foods that have an alkaline reaction, such as fruits and vegetables.

Dr. Lucius M. Bush, in his book *The Secret of Sinusitis and Headaches*, suggests massaging the side wall of the nasal passage to relieve congestion, to open up the nasal passage.

It is thought that emotional damage, not just bacterial infection, can trigger sinus headache.

Good circulation, warm feet, no constipation and a non-mucous forming diet are the essentials in sinusitis treatment.

Substituting soy bean milk for cow's milk helps to restore the sinuses to healthy functioning. Cow's milk is mucous-forming.

To relieve the pressure, the opening must be cleared and drainage encouraged. Hot and cold packs (alternately) on the face and forehead help in this opening process.

Treatment for sinutis should begin with an enema. Then regulate bowel elimination to three good evacuations a day. The only cure is to thoroughly cleanse the body of all toxic poisons.

A fruit-juice diet for four or five days, drinking all you can, is stressed. One kind of fruit a day. Do not mix the juices. Orange, grapefruit, lemon, pineapple, or grape juice should be alternated each day.

Herbs recommended for sinusitis are plantain, golden seal, elderberry flowers, Rocky Mountain grape root, marshmallow root, fennel seed, hops, yellow dock, burdock root and red clover blossoms.

It is recommended that certain herbs be smoked to relieve the distress of sinus infection. Such herbs are cubeb berries, peach tree leaves, peppermint leaves and mullein leaves.

Supplements are of prime importance in the treatment of sinusitis. Vitamin C and B-12 are especially stressed. Also two teaspoonfuls apple cider vinegar and two teaspoonfuls honey in a glass of water. Calcium, phosphorus and vitamins A and D are also advocated. Bonemeal, vitamins A and D, raw liver or desiccated liver, and 300 mgs of vitamin C from rosehips used every day, has proved very effective.

SKIN DISORDERS

Ringworm or Impetigo

Peroxide applied to either ringworm or impetigo is effective. A salve made by mixing powdered sulphur and lard together and adding one teaspoon of lemon juice is also good.

For internal use drink a tea made from golden seal, hops, boneset or plantain.

Erysipelas

For erysipelas, bathe parts with a solution made with golden seal, lobelia, burdock, yellow dock and myrrh. Powdered slippery elm bark sprinkled on is also recommended.

Eczema

Eczema has cleared up when the diet was made adequate and especially rich in linoleic acid and all the B vitamins. Some cases were helped when vegetable oil was given. Eczema has cleared up like magic with corn oil. A dose of one tablespoonful was given and increased gradually until four tablespoonfuls were taken three times a day.

Stubborn cases of psoriasis usually disappear rapidly when vegetable oil and lecithin are added to the diet. Another recommended remedy for psoriasis is 36 grams of lecithin daily; gradually decrease until 4 grams daily, which should be continued as a maintenance dose.

An application of apple cider vinegar is said to be helpful.

POISON OAK OR IVY

First let us consider eradicating this pest. A solution of calcium chlorate (½lb to the gallon of water) sprayed on when it is in full leaf. Results are better if done on a warm, sunny day. However, it will kill any vegetation with which it comes in contact. This solution is not poisonous to animals. It does not kill large trees and shrubs unless it is sprayed directly on them.

For the agonizing itching of poison oak or ivy, make a solution of equal parts of a strong tea of white oak bark and lime water. Apply saturated bandage.

Make a strong tea of spearmint, peach tree leaves, plantain, lobelia or golden seal and apply to the area.

Drink chestnut leaf tea several times a day and also apply frequently to the rash.

Every time it itches, rub golden rod leaves, in cold water and bathe parts. Allow to dry for itself.

A strong solution of epsom salts is also recommended.

If you think you have come in contact with these pests, bathe exposed parts with vinegar.

HIVES

Hives are believed to be due to lack of power of the liver to kill off harmful organisms. The following herb teas are

E

recommended. Sassafrass bark, red clover blossoms, bull nettle and yarrow.

Most skin disorders will respond readily to herb teas.

BITES AND STINGS

There are certain odours and substances which most insects dislike. Oil of citronella, oil of geranium or oil of eucalyptus are useful for rubbing on exposed parts of the body.

For bee stings, remove the sting and apply bruised green leaf of plantain. Relief is almost instantaneous.

For bee stings, wet soap, moistened baking soda or weak ammonia. For wasp stings, use vinegar or lemon juice. Raw potato or damp earth are also good for wasp stings. Aloes is an old French remedy for bee or wasp stings.

For most insect bites, especially mosquito bites, use wet soap or weak ammonia. For spider bites use vinegar or ammonia.

The following is said to be effective for mad dog bites. Take raw onions, green garden rue, salt and powdered elecampane root. Beat well together and apply to wound.

Plinius, the Roman naturalist, believed that garlic is an excellent remedy for mad dog bite, to be eaten and also applied to the wound.

For snake bite, the pioneers wet saltpetre with a little water and applied it to the bite. A sack of common table salt was also dampened and laid over the bite. Lobelia is a valuable herb to be applied and also *very* small doses taken internally. *Lobelia should be used only by a good practitioner.* These are to be used for emergencies until help can be had.

Oil of Peppermint is cooling to bee stings or insect bites.

Bees working on flowers rarely sting unless molested.

STOMACH DISORDERS

The stomach comes in for its share of discomfort and distress. The many anti-acids advertised in magazine and on television attest to the thousands of stomach sufferers.

Anti-acids are not the answer. The only sure relief for this troublesome ailment is found in safe herbal demulcents which coat the irritated membranes throughout the digestive tract.

Slippery elm bark is one of the best demulcents in the vegetable kingdom. It has a soothing influence on the stomach and intestines. It is superior to whole milk in its ability to neutralize stomach acids.

Okra will also protect the sensitive duodenal surfaces and relieve distress.

The carminative action of garlic helps and arrests formation of gas and fermentation of food.

A glass of milk two hours after each meal will absorb the extra acid which the stomach pours out in periods of stress. Goat's milk is especially curative and healing to the stomach.

Wild cherry bark tea is good for a sour stomach.

Hops have been a long-standing remedy for stomach ailments.

For gas on the stomach, one teaspoonful of caraway seed to a cup of boiling water is helpful.

One-half cupful of pennyroyal tea is good for a sick stomach. Pennyroyal should never be taken during pregnancy, NEVER. Calamus root will stop cramp in the stomach. A tea of golden seal is one of the best stomach remedies known. Sarsaparilla is also a good stomach remedy, as well as "life everlasting", camomile and peppermint.

Peppermint, calamus, gentian and golden seal make one of the best formulae for indigestion.

Papaya juice and also papaya tea are an excellent stomach remedy. I have found that peppermint combined with papaya is especially good.

A combination of golden seal, German cheese plant, camomile and slippery elm bark can help in acid stomach and ulcers of the stomach. Shepherd's purse will stop bleeding from stomach ulcers in fifteen minutes.

SYPHILIS AND GONORRHOEA

Syphilis and gonorrhea are not the same thing. Each is caused by a different germ. One may have both diseases at the same time. They are both social diseases and many times treatment is not sought because of shame.

It is advisable to seek orthodox medical treatment for these conditions.

TUBERCULOSIS

When the system is nutritionally perfect, tubercle bacillus or any other germ can have no effect on a person.

A Californian doctor supplemented the diet of twenty terminal cases in an out-clinic experiment with natural foods. Many were started back to health in one year's time.

Calmette Guerin, an anti-tuberculosis vaccine has not proved effective.

It has been suggested that babies be innoculated with BCG as a matter of course. An 8-month old boy died a few days after an innoculation. The autopsy showed the cause of death to be widespread tuberculosis.

In spite of the increased use of anti-TB drugs, TB has continued to increase at a rapid rate each year.

Wood betony and wood sage have been used for TB. A wineglass full of the tea was taken three times a day. Comfrey is also said to be an effective treatment.

Herbs have helped so many in fighting disease. Yet learned doctors say there is no scientific proof.

In the face of such contrary evidence, we can know for ourselves of the outstanding virtues of harmless herbs.

VARICOSE VEINS

Varicose veins are the result of stagnation of blood in the veins and the consequent weakening of the walls and valves. Prolonged standing is highly undesirable. However, brisk walking is favourable.

Lay on your back and elevate the legs, draining the blood from the legs to relieve pressure. Bathe legs with cold water to tone and strengthen the tissues.

Tight garters should never be worn.

A good diet will strengthen the tissues and keep the legs free from varicose veins.

WHOOPING COUGH

Ephedrin (MaHuang) boiled in water and administered for whooping cough is an old remedy.

Make a syrup of one ounce of chestnut leaves, half ounce black cohosh, quarter ounce lobelia, one ounce coltsfoot and a pinch of cayenne. One teaspoonful is taken every hour or as needed. I gave this recipe to my children. In about two weeks they were free from whooping. Other children in the community who received shots were still whooping most of the summer.

A study of the blood of whooping-cough patients showed that the normal acid balance is upset. Baking soda will neutralize the acid.

To one pint of boiling water add a pinch of cayenne, one slice of lemon, three tablespoonfuls of honey and one ounce of shredded slippery elm bark. Allow to steep one-half hour. Take frequently in small doses. This is also a good remedy.

CHAPTER V

How the Glands Work

I T is impossible to say that any one of the functions of the body is dependent entirely on any single one of the glands because of their interrelationship one with another.

The adrenals, located just in front of the kidneys, are a source of adrenalin. Adrenalin is released into the bloodstream under stress of any kind, such as fright, anger, pain, heat, cold, fatigue, shock, etc. Exhaustion of the adrenal gland occurs in severe burns.

Since stress plays such an important part in the adrenals, the emotions should be kept under control at all times if the glands are to function properly.

There is an abundance of vitamin C in healthy adrenals. However, vitamin C is not alone in the essentials of the adrenals. It takes all of the vitamins and minerals that constitute good nutrition if the adrenals are to function normally.

The thyroid gland is located in the throat in front of and on either side of the windpipe.

There is scarcely a tissue in the body that can remain in optimum health without the influence of the thyroid.

The calcium balance of the body is closely associated with this gland. The thyroid influences the nervous system, the motion of the intestinal track, the acid-alkaline balance of the blood, the circulatory system, storage and distribution of fat. Many obese persons are suffering from a thyroid imbalance.

Degrees of sluggishness in an individual are apparent in proportion to a thyroid deficiency.

There is research being done which suggests that some of the coronary difficulties may be associated with the thyroid.

The most important element in the health of the thyroid is iodine. Kelp and all seafoods are rich in iodine. Complete food supplements contain enough iodine for the daily intake.

The thyroid is a sort of accelerator to the rest of the glands. It regulates the action of every cell and has much to do with the speed with which nourishment is taken up by the blood. The hormone manufactured by the thyroid has been likened to a whip that speeds up the various functions of the body.

A goitre is a chronic enlargement of the thyroid gland. It is a visible sign of iodine shortage.

Eat more iodine-rich fish, seaweeds such as kelp and Irish moss. Also step up your intake of vitamin B foods. Together, iodine and vitamin B will correct abnormalcy of the thyroid gland activity that simple goitre implies.

When the thyroid is subnormal, the body cannot use its nitrogenous food. This unassimilated material is then stored in the tissues in the form of deposits of mucous material.

There are also symptoms of calcium deficiency in goitre.

Thyroxine is the secretion of the thyroid gland. It is made from iodine and the amino acid called tyrosine. The thyroid also needs riboflavin to manufacture thyroxine.

Under no circumstances should the thyroid be removed. If the thyroid is not functioning normally or goitre is present, treat the condition by natural means. A well-rounded, fully adequate diet, pure water augmented with harmless herb teas, should be considered. Iodine in the form of kelp or other seaweeds should be used. Never take inorganic iodine such as iodized salt.

The parathyroid glands are associated with the thyroid gland. They are so important that without them life would be impossible. When the parathyroids are not nourished properly, the hands become unsteady and palsy develops. This is due especially to a lack of magnesium. The nails and hair also become brittle.

The pituitary gland is about the size of a pea and is located at the base of the brain. It is often referred to as the master gland. It is really two glands, the front and the back pituitary, also called lobes. Each of these secretes several hormones which have different functions.

The pituitary supervises the functions of the other glands and of each cell in the body. To function harmoniously, the pituitary requires especially manganese and the whole of the B complex.

The pancreas is probably the least understood of the glands in the body.

It has been learned through clinical demonstration that long-continued inflammation will eventually cause irritation of the liver and gall bladder. For this reason, irrespective of the treatment given to the liver or gall bladder, the condition will not respond to treatment until the pancreas is treated.

The small end of the pancreas deals with the manufacture of insulin. When there is an insufficient supply of insulin, which maintains a normal blood sugar level, diabetes will result.

When the pancreas is not functioning properly, no carbohydrates or sugar should be eaten. Beverages should be fruit and vegetable juices and herb teas.

CHAPTER VI

Your White Bloodstream

THE lymph is a clear, colourless fluid which bathes and permeates the solid structure of the body. It has been estimated that in the body of an adult there may be thirty to forty pints of lymph compared with twelve to fourteen pints of blood.

The main function of the lymph system is to carry off poisonous wastes resulting from metabolism.

The circulation of this lymphatic fluid is a slow one compared with the circulation of the blood. The lymph passes along the lymphatic system by a sort of suction action caused by the difference in blood pressure between that of the arteries which supply the lymph to the cells and the pressure of the veins which receive it after it has been cleansed and rid of its waste.

This difference is regulated by the secretions of certain glands. The thyroid and the suprarenals are the most important of these.

When the lymphatic system does not do its work properly, congestion sets in.

The lymph does its work of collecting and removing waste by a set of tubes called lymphatics. These tubes or ducts unite again and again to form about twenty main lines for each limb. Each line or trunk extends upward and most of them unite to form the thoracic duct. This duct lies upon the spinal column and extends into the neck where it opens into a large vein.

At regular intervals the lymphs open into small, bag-like bodies filled with cells. Each of these is called a lymph gland or node. The lymph flows through these nodes, where it is filtered. The lymph nodes may be felt in the neck, groins and armpits. In the case of inflammation or congestion, these nodes swell and sometimes break down.

About two quarts of lymph passes through the thoracic duct daily, where it mingles with the blood.

Our health and even our lives depend on the perfect functioning of this intricate system.

This filter system traps anything potentially harmful. The lymph nodes strain out these wastes and destroy them. Normally, this filtering process is so efficient that the blood is rendered clean and free from invading organisms. The lymphatic system also produces antibodies which destroy harmful bacteria. When infection sets in, the lymphatic system produces thousands of white cells which fight the infection.

It is certain that if we do not furnish needed nourishment so the lymphatics can carry it to the cells and do its work of filtering out waste, and we overwork and overload this intricate network with chemicals, poisons, etc., disease is sure to follow.

Pure, wholesome food and herbs alone can assist in this marvellous work which goes on so efficiently that we are not aware of its performance.

CHAPTER VII

Refreshing Sleep Without Drugs

MORE than 6,000,000 persons take sleeping pills to go to sleep each night.

Many sleeping aids are advertised as harmless and non-habit-forming. But are they really?

The casual user becomes more and more tense. It becomes more difficult to get to sleep each night. The tension mounts with continued use.

Tension is a dangerous thing. It interferes with the various processes of the body. The body must be repaired and recharged. Energy is stored by the body during sleep. Much of the toxic poisons that accumulate in the body go through a process of elimination while we sleep.

Sleep is the result of the gradual withdrawal of the blood from the brain. Nervous tension causes a surplus amount of blood to circulate in the cerebral region.

Soaking the feet in hot water will draw the blood from the head.

Sleeping pills are not necessary. If your diet is right, you will sleep like a baby without that harmful crutch.

Cutting down on salt in the diet will relieve sleeplessness.

Lack of calcium contributes to sleeplessness. Instead of taking the advertised sleep-aids, increase your calcium intake.

Another helpful suggestion is to stretch. Take a good stretch, one that you can feel all along your spine, and you will sleep like a kitten. I have followed this idea many times. It works.

The herbal kingdom holds sedatives that are sure to help and are definitely harmless.

One such sedative formula consists of skullcap, lady's slipper, catnip and valerian. Take it hot at bedtime.

A tea made with hops and skullcap is also a good nightcap. Camomile tea is also good to induce sleep.

Don't cheat yourself on sleep. Invite restful sleep the harmless way. Go to bed at a regular time each night. Start slowing down an hour or so before your regular bedtime. Avoid heavy eating before you go to bed.

When you find yourself battling with the demons of insomnia, take a harmless herbal calmative. Try stretching and relax and sleep.

CHAPTER VIII

Female Disorders

THE generative organs of a woman are vital to her well-being.

From the time those organs being to function and the little girl crosses the threshold into womanhood until the cessation of the menstrual flow, a woman may find peace and joy of living or experience distress, discomfort or downright suffering.

The healthy performance of the functioning of the female organs is essential to good health. No derangement in these functions can exist for any length of time without drawing the entire life of the individual into sympathetic suffering.

In the case of young girls, the flow may be scanty and irregular. At this time it is not wise to give medicine to promote the secretion beyond attention to warm clothing, according to the temperature, and a good diet, avoiding tea and coffee and highly seasoned foods. This will generally be sufficient to produce a normal flow. If, however, there is abnormal pain at this time, one teaspoon of camomile flowers in a cup of boiling water and sipped warm, but not hot, will be helpful. A tea made of equal parts of horehound and raspberry leaves will produce a normal flow. Life root is equally good. Spikenard is helpful in cases of suppressed menstruation.

A woman must at all times keep herself free from constipation. There are herbs that can be taken for constipation. However, it is my opinion that a proper diet will do more to relieve constipation than any laxative and is much better for a person. Never take anything but a herbal laxative.

Pain in the heels of females may be the only evidence of ovarian abscess. Pain and swelling of the breasts will evince some trouble in the same side of the uterus or fallopian tube.

Knee-chest position is a preventive and cure of pelvic

diseases in women. Rock back and forth while standing on knees and elbows.

An excessive flow of blood from the womb during menstruation is one of the most frequent complaints of women. Herbs recommended are red raspberry leaves and black haw.

Herbs for cramp are camomile, valerian, skullcap, lady's slipper. Red clover blossoms and sweet flag are also good. Cramp bark is especially good.

A good female tonic consists of equal parts of black cohosh, star root (aletris farinosa), motherwort, black haw and camomile.

Women whose liver is not functioning normally are likely to experience menstrual difficulties and pain.

Menstruation is thought to drain vitamin C and perhaps vitamin P from the system.

Blood calcium falls during the week prior to menstruation. This causes nervousness, irritability and depression. Further drop at onset of flow causes cramp of the muscular walls of the uterus. Additional calcium should be taken, also vitamin D.

Easing premenstrual tension is important. Camomile is excellent for hysterical and nervous afflictions of women.

There is a tremendous impact on a woman's whole system at the cessation of the menstrual flow.

At middle-age, production of estrogen begins to fail, followed by cessation of the menstrual cycle. It is at this time that there are changes in body metabolism. Dosage with synthetic estrogen is not the answer. It can even prove harmful. It prolongs the menopause. A harmless herbal sedative is all that is needed. If a woman will take the following herbal tonic at this time, much discomfort and suffering can be avoided. Black cohosh, sweet flag, liquorice root, star root (aletris farinosa), black haw, cramp bark (viburnum opulus), squaw-weed (false valerian, also called female regulator) and motherwort. One cup during the day, mostly with meals, is recommended.

Liquorice in a female remedy has female hormone action. The herbs helionas and alteris farinosa have also been found to contain estrogen.

My favourite sedative, catnip, valerian, camomile, skullcap, lady slipper and peppermint, is all that is needed during the menopause outside of good nutrition.

Headache and nervousness are also due to a toxic condition of the body during the menopause.

The change of life should be a natural change. It should hold no fear for a healthy well-nourished woman.

A good herbal tonic to be taken during the menopause is a combination of golden seal, motherwort, pullsatilla, arrach, tansy, black haw and valerian.

I would again stress the importance of a good diet. The best results of botanic drugs can be obtained only when the diet is of the best quality. Herbs can help in any condition, but it takes longer for nature to do her part in the healing process if the body is in a toxic condition from improper foods or the lack of essential food factors.

CHAPTER IX

Pregnancy and Delivery

CHILD-BIRTH should be a fine, fearless experience. It is true there may be some discomfort even bordering on distress. During pregnancy, the whole glandular system is overactive. This may cause some distress. However, if a woman will keep herself well-nourished, there should be no real cause for alarm.

Peach tree leaves are useful to curb vomiting or morning sickness in early pregnancy. It is also slightly laxative.

The diet of expectant mothers in a certain village was closely supervised. The diet consisted of raw milk, butter, eggs, Cheshire cheese, oatmeal, broth, salad in abundance, meat and wholemeal bread to which raw wheat germ was added. The mothers were usually able to nurse their babies. Pulmonary diseases were almost unknown among the babies. One of the striking features was the happy personality of the children.

Lack of vitamin K may produce abortion. Patients treated with synthetic vitamin K for this purpose do not respond as they should. Doctors using synthetic vitamin K for abortion have caused a disease known as Kernicterus which results in spasticity and mental retardation of the child.

Alfalfa and peppermint teas are good to prevent abortion. Star root (aletris farinosa) is the best botanical known to avert abortion. Vitamin P has also been found to be a preventive. The best source of vitamin P is found together with vitamin C in rosehips.

Smoking has been shown to be detrimental to an easy, normal delivery. The mother-to-be owes it to herself and her baby to keep herself under such control.

An investigator for the American Heart Association warned that expectant mothers should be given 'flu shots. Most

F

vaccines used to combat Asian 'flu produce antibodies which clash with blood type A.

Giving the mother anaesthesia in childbirth may result in birth injuries. The mother is not able to labour with her full strength. The doctor must then manipulate the position of the emerging infant, frequently tugging with great force and pulling the head into an abnormally strained position. This can cause a slight malpositioning of the head and affect the spinal vertebrae. The injury may not be obvious, but it creates enough arterial pressure to prevent the brain from functioning at its best.

It has also been found that interference in the birth process by the attendant deprives the baby of oxygen during childbirth. One of the major causes of cerebral palsy is a lack of oxygen to the baby in difficult and prolonged labour.

There should be no X-ray examination either on the man or woman two months before impregnation—and definitely should not be allowed at any time during pregnancy.

The best protective agent the pregnant woman has against the possibility her child will be born deformed is a high consumption of the B complex vitamins. A survey of top authorities reveals that B complex prevents birth deformities. Vitamin E and A are also recommended. A full complement of all the vitamins and minerals is, of course, best.

The physician should know the essential ingredients of all drugs he administers during pregnancy. There should be a ban placed on the use of all drugs by expectant mothers, especially in early pregnancy. This would be the only safe course to prevent another thalidomide catastrophe.

Clamping the umbilical cord before a newborn infant has drawn his second breath has been thought to be a factor in the development of what the doctors call "respiratory distress syndrome" or possible fatal breathing difficulty.

The complications of childbirth are often the result of teenage malnutrition. Inadequate physical development, especially of the female pelvis, or a derangement of its structure, creates a crowded environment for foetal development and a restricted passage for normal childbirth.

The suffering of childbirth could be minimized or eliminated entirely and a natural, normal birth be experienced if certain herb teas were taken the last six weeks of pregnancy. I know this to be true. Many pregnant women have taken these herbs and have experienced unusual results.

One young woman in particular is built so that a difficult delivery was anticipated. With her first baby the doctor did not feel it was necessary for him to hurry to wash up. The baby was born before he was ready. In less than an hour after she entered the hospital, the baby was born and she was cleaned up and back in bed. Such a delivery would prevent childbirth injury due to prolonged delivery.

This same young woman had a similar experience when her second child was born. Her second delivery was so unusual that the doctor called it miraculous. The nurse in attendance told me that my young friend had only two hard pains and the baby was born.

There are a number of herbs that can be taken for easy childbirth. A teaspoon of the herb or mixed herbs to a cup of boiling water and one cup a day should be taken, a mouthful at a time.

Spikenard and red raspberry leaves are exceptionally good when taken during the last six weeks of pregnancy. This is what I suggest. Hot tansy tea taken to increase labour pains is beneficial. Black cohosh taken two or three months before confinement is also good. Blue cohosh taken one or two weeks before confinement is also good. Three tablespoonfuls of the tea made of sow thistle taken in wine is said to make delivery so easy and speedy that the woman is able to walk about shortly afterwards with no feeling of weakness or distress.

Music has been used to sooth patients in labour. Of thirty women who received musicotherapy during childbirth, all but three found it helpful.

Many mothers experience painful caked breast. This too can be helped with herbs. Take a handful of elderberry blossoms and simmer in grease or oil in a covered dish in a slow oven. Strain and apply warm. This will help every time.

Fennel seed boiled in barley water is said to be good for

mothers who wish to nurse their babies. It increases the milk supply. This tea is harmless and so much better than shop tea, with its high tannin content, which is suggested by doctors.

Lactating women must have a sufficient supply of vitamin B to stimulate secretion of milk and transmit as much as possible to the baby.

CHAPTER X

Babies and their Care

You have an important choice to make when your newborn comes to stay. Either you will breast feed your baby or put him on the bottle. It is being stressed again today that breast feeding is a must for babies.

Successful breast feeding has definite advantages for both you and your baby. Doctors are certain now that breast-fed babies show higher resistance to intestinal disorders. 90% of deaths from intestinal disorders occur in bottle-fed babies.

An article in *Science Magazine* for August 1962 gave specific evidence of the value of mother's milk in fighting dangerous infection, especially staphylococcus aureus (staph).

Many other advantages of breast feeding include greater resistance to infectious colds and a better adjustment in later life. Also a new disease, retrolental fibrophasia, is far less frequent among breast-fed babies.

Your ability to nurse your baby is largely a matter which you may determine and even regulate. You must believe in nursing and in your ability to nurse.

It usually requires about two weeks to become accustomed to breast feeding. You should not stop nursing just because you encounter difficulties.

Human milk is richer in vitamin A than cows' milk. So the bottle-fed baby does not get as much vitamin A as he needs unless he is given a supplement.

It is said that a mother can adequately nourish her baby on nothing more than breast milk for six months.

It has been found that women who nurse their babies are less liable to develop breast cancer.

If you must bottle feed your baby, the following is a good nourishing formula. Whole milk or soy milk, honey and slippery elm bark (powdered). Honey is valuable in bottle feeding. It requires no further digestion. It contains minerals and vitamins. It is also a valuable help in overcoming constipation. If you are not able to breast feed your baby, goat's milk is one of the best substitutes. An infant will really thrive on it.

When it comes time for solid or semi-solid food, be certain that the food you give your baby has adequate nutrients and also that it has no injurious ingredients.

Babies fed a certain baby food either died or were rendered cripples. The formula was corrected. The newer formula, while it has lower amounts, still contains harmful amounts of Fluorine.

Milk formulae cannot always be depended upon either. One formula often prescribed for babies caused convulsions in the infants. The cause of the seizures was finally found to be a deficiency in B–6. A new sterilization process adopted by the company reduced the B–6 level, a vitamin which is susceptible to heat.

You cannot be too careful. Your baby is the most precious gift you could ever be given. Be certain that the feeding of your baby is adequate, pure and dependable.

A baby may gain slowly during the first five weeks. Too rapid gains in weight above six ounces a week are not advisable, except in cases of a very undernourished baby. A healthy baby should double its weight by five or six months, and treble it by the end of the first year. Fat babies may appear to be good babies, but they are really sluggish and slow to respond to external stimuli.

Too rich milk kill's baby's appetite.

Massage may help baby to overcome constipation.

Soy milk has been found to be nourishing for babies and children. Goat milk is also recommended.

A healthy baby is not cross when cutting teeth. Restless, fretful, teething babies need more calcium and vitamin D. The first teeth should appear at six months. The baby should have six teeth at one year, twelve at a year and a half and sixteen at two years.

If baby is fretful when teething, or is colicy, a weak, warm tea made from either catnip, camomile, elder flowers, peppermint or fennel seed will be beneficial.

Fretful babies used to be given paregoric, which is really camphorated tincture of opium.

The Choctaw Indians boiled the root of spikenard in water and gave it to peevish babies, which is absolutely harmless.

By four months a baby should be able to hold up his head. From three to five months he usually begins to laugh aloud. At seven or eight months he may sit erect and soon will begin to creep and should begin to walk from twelve to eighteen months. At one year he usually can speak a few words. At eight or nine months he should be bright, slim and active. The best-fed children are the brightest.

The fruit of the carob tree, also called St. John's bread, has been made into a medicine which is helping modern babies recover from diarrhoea. Babies given carob flour in water every four hours were cured in about one-third the time it took babies treated in the same way but not getting the carob flour.

For infants who cannot urinate, watermelon seed tea has long been known to be beneficial.

Babies who have difficulty digesting cow's milk are said to be relieved by the addition of powdered apple to the milk. Tests showed that cow's milk is lower in acidity than human breast milk, which is the cause of the digestive problem.

Pediatricians prescribe orange juice for babies as a matter of routine. From the *Journal of Pediatrics* (October 1953) we learn that orange juice is slow to digest and can cause real distress. An article in *JAMA* (May 21, 1960) tells of evidence of violent reactions to citrus juices.

Never force oily substances on a baby. Pneumonia (lipoid pneumonia) may be caused by oily substances being drawn into the lungs if the child does not swallow properly, especially if he resists it.

Boric acid is often used to bathe the eyes and in baby powders. Evidence shows that boric acid can be very toxic and actually cause death, even when applied externally. It may be absorbed through the broken skin or mucous membrane. The lungs, kidneys, bladder, brain, liver and intestines have been found to be badly damaged in cases where boric acid, or boric acid containing powders, were used on infants.

Today it is thought necessary to inoculate babies with vaccines and various other shots.

Babies are born with a natural immunity to disease which should last six months. The thymus gland is responsible for this defence against disease. The cells in the thymus gland travel to the spleen at birth and become lymphoid cells. These cells produce fighting antibodies. After six months, the body manufactures interferon as a defence against disease. It must, however, be produced in sufficient amounts. If the body receives all the food factors necessary, and such things as refined products, cokes, ice cream (commercial) and candy are withheld, interferon will be produced in sufficient amounts. Drugs of any kind interfere with the production of interferon. Aspirin especially is harmful to interferon production. It has become a common practice to give infants aspirin because advertising says it is the thing to do.

That is the way God made us. Today, when so much is known about feeding babies, why should God's way be tampered with?

It is an established scientific fact that the widespread use of vaccines among the general public cannot be justified.

An abundance of fresh air is one of baby's greatest needs. It increases resistance to disease, strengthens recuperative powers, improves the appetite and aids digestion.

Whenever your baby shows signs of coming down with any illness, the first thing to do is to open the bowels. Give the small patient a warm catnip tea enema. Much illness can be averted in this way.

Remember, it is easier to keep a baby well than to make him well after illness has set in.

CHAPTER XI

The Care of Older Children

IN a Toronto Children's Hospital, increasing numbers of cases of premature puberty were found. The sight of a child with two fully developed breasts and other signs of female maturity was not uncommon.

According to an article in *The Toronto Star* (January 18, 1964), it has been found that cosmetics may contain powerful sex hormones than can be absorbed through a child's skin. Just a casual contact with these ingredients in a cosmetic grandma uses could be the cause of what is termed "pseudo-puberty".

Stammering is a bad handicap. Most cured stammerers are self-cured. The stammerer has only to forget his speech difficulty. Stammering cannot be cured by an outside influence such as prescriptions or directions from a physician. A stammerer will not stammer when his attention is removed from the problem of uttering words. Thus he will not stammer while singing, repeating poetry, imitating another's voice or when his attention is distracted in other ways. Chewing-speaking exercises is one form of treatment.

Nervous mothers who are always fretting about whether a baby or small child eats enough are likely to have nervous children who stutter.

Never force food upon a child. If he is hungry he will eat. If he is not hungry, forcing him to eat may upset his digestive processes. Be certain though that his lack of appetite is not due to piecing between meals on poorly chosen snacks.

In toilet training, do it with love. Give the child a feeling of security. Harsh methods will produce a spirit of retaliation and hatred.

Never lift a young child by his arms. The ligaments may be sprained by such treatment.

The familiar "Don't scratch it!" is often heard when a youngster has insect bites or poison ivy. Scratching properly done will do no damage. Itching of a bite or ivy poisoning can be relieved by soft rubbing with the palm of the hand, (not the fingernails) around the affected area, not directly over it.

Rickets is not only a disease of infants. It may occur up to fourteen years of age. This ailment results from a vitamin D deficiency. However, vitamin D requires calcium and phosphorus to be effective. A growing child needs at least five grams of calcium per day. One quart of milk contains only one gram. If babies are slow to walk, correct the diet.

Children's diseases are mostly of the eruptive type. They are merely a toxic system trying to rid itself of impurities.

For measles, either saffron flowers, elder flowers, catnip, camomile or rosemary tea, taken hot, will break out the rash and check the fever. Three tablespoonfuls of the herb to a quart of water, and boiled down to one pint, is the way to prepare the tea.

In spite of inoculation today for measles and mumps, these diseases are still with us.

Hot catnip tea helps to relieve the pain of mumps. Saffron is good in cases of scarlet fever.

For diphtheria, pineapple juice, lemon juice and honey, or cider vinegar and honey, have been effective. A pinch of cayenne may be added for older children. Pineapple juice will cut the mucous.

In cases of croup, make the child perspire with warm herb teas and a hot-water bottle. Elderberry flowers, peppermint and honey are good.

Colds and 'flu can be treated with a mild tea made from catnip, elderberry flowers and peppermint leaves. For a baby, I used one teaspoonful every half hour. Sage tea is also good for adults.

Elder flowers are good in cases of constipation. Give your child figs for constipation.

Stinging nettle tea is a good tonic for children.

Herb teas, harmless, effective remedies, are helpful in all children's diseases.

Grated raw apple sprinkled with anise seed in a salad will get rid of worms. Cold sage tea is also good for worms. Remember always to give a mild laxative before breakfast following any worm treatment.

A backward child was given vitamin E. The parents had been told their child would be slower and have weaker muscles than the average child. The diagnosis was congenital hypotonia. After taking 50 mg of vitamin E in small doses, per day for two weeks, the child showed marvellous improvement.

Needless tonsillectomies have and are still being performed. The tonsils are part of the family of lymph glands. They are located on either side of the passage from the mouth to the pharynx. They were placed there by an all-wise creator and were meant to last a lifetime. They are important little chemical laboratories which aid in waste disposal.

The tonsils have important protective functions of self-vaccination or immunization, especially in the very persons, our children, from whom they are so wantonly removed. It is now recognised that the tonsils are especially active in produ cing anti-toxins against acute diseases. Removing them breaks down the body's natural defence.

Diseased tonsils respond to treatment just as easily as any abnormal condition in the body. There is no such thing as tonsils too diseased to save. Tonsil removal is so much propaganda.

A well-known physician and surgeon admitted that of 2,500 tonsillectomies he performed, there were none so far gone but what could have been saved by proper treatment.

For prevention and restoration of infected tonsils, provide a wholesome, balanced diet, excluding all white flour products, white sugar, cokes, candy and ice cream (commercial). Tasty meals, desserts and delicacies just as tempting to the small-fry can be provided without these worthless refined and harmful trash.

An investigation of the removal of tonsils (thirty to sixty days before an epidemic of infantile paralysis occurs) showed more attacks and more severe attacks among those whose tonsils were recently removed.

Every part of the body has a function or work to perform. Removing one part does not remedy the condition.

When a child feels the slightest difficulty in swallowing, whether it is because of a mild sore throat or a more severe case of engorged tonsils or diphtheria, stop all solid food. And as I have stressed many times in this book, first give a herb tea enema. Catnip is good. Pineapple juice is the best remedy, letting the juice trickle slowly down to bathe the inflamed throat and tonsils. Crushed pineapple, canned without sugar, is also good. Vegetable juices are valuable in removing waste.

Wring from cold water (not ice cold) four thicknesses of muslin or a piece of terry cloth, sufficiently large to encircle the neck. Cover this with a dry cloth. Allow to remain on for several hours or over night. Repeat as necessary. And remember, keep the bowels open, beginning with a warm catnip tea enema.

Children should seldom be given medicine in the same doses recommended for adults. The usual proportionate dose, where the medicine is suitable for a child, is as follows:

> 4 years—one-sixth adult dose
> 6 ,, —one-fourth adult dose
> 8 ,, —one-third adult dose
> 12 ,, —one-half adult dose
> 15 ,, —two-thirds adult dose

CHAPTER XII

Beauty Secrets

ARE you satisfied with what your mirror tells you? If not, do something about it. Don't expect dramatic improvement though. Damage done by years of neglect and improper skin care cannot be erased in minutes. Beware of cosmetic advertisements that would have you believe such claims. Today women spend approximately $750,000,000 a year on cosmetics.

You cannot push back the years, but you can be attractive at any age. If you know how to care for your health, you can attain the kind of beauty which does not fade with the years, for it is ageless.

The first step in beauty care is a thorough cleansing from within. A clean alimentary tract is your best beauty insurance.

Food has an important influence on your complexion.

An incident as told in the Bible shows what an effect the food we eat has on the condition of the skin.

King Nebuchadnezzar chose four Hebrew boys to teach them the language and learning of the Chaldeans. The boys chose to not eat the food on the king's table. They asked to be given only "pulse and water". Webster says that pulse may be any edible seeds or grains or the plant yielding the same. It was agreed that such would be their fare for ten days. At the end of that time they were compared with those who ate the king's rich food and found that "Their countenances appeared fairer and fatter in flesh than all the children which did eat the king's meat".

The choice of a sensible diet can do wonders for your skin. A diet high in vitamins and minerals will give your skin a bloom and texture which no cosmetics can. Without these essential factors your skin will be muddy and dull looking.

All green leafy vegetables, including herb teas, are recognized as excellent sources of vitamins and minerals. Dandelion greens are nature's best beauty treatment. The leaves of this lawn pest are literally a gold-mine of vitamin A. Rough, scaly skin may be a sign of vitamin A deficiency. These greens also contain riboflavin, the lack of which may cause large pores and black heads. Wrinkles around the lips may be caused by an extreme riboflavin deficiency. Dandelions are also rich in vitamin C, which is needed to help the blood carry oxygen to the skin cells.

Insufficient protein can bring about ageing with amazing speed, allowing lines and wrinkles to appear.

Salt is the worst thing a woman can use because it causes a drying out of the skin and can lead to wrinkles.

Experiments have proved that in women who eliminate white sugar from their diets, the lines of their faces took on a much more handsome appearance. A diet top-heavy in starches and sugars is acid-forming and ageing.

Excessive indulgence in fats and starches, pastries and gravies and highly seasoned foods clouds the skin and robs it of vital beauty. Replace chocolate, cocoa and greasy foods for two weeks with alfalfa tea and see the difference in your complexion.

Lack of essential vitamins and minerals is expressed in a muddy, pasty complexion. Menus packed with vitamins and minerals will give you a skin you can be proud of.

Carrots, if eaten raw or juiced, will give a complexion no cosmetic can boast of, will give a ruddy glow to the cheeks no rouge in the world can give.

Freckles show that the adrenals are large and poorly nourished. When these glands are properly nourished, the freckles tend to disappear. To remove freckles, obtain fresh elder flowers. Cover with cold water. Rain water or distilled water is best. If this is not obtainable, boil water one hour, then let it get cold. After covering well with water, allow to stand overnight. Strain and use to bathe the freckles morning and night. Also, chickweed mashed in soft water and apply the mash to the freckles.

The protective acid mantle of the skin is destroyed by the use of harsh alkaline soaps. Soap irritates the natural acid base of the skin. It is made mostly from caustic alkalies and fats which penetrate the skin's protective layer and leach out the skin's protective emulsion.

This acid mantle of the skin is spoken of as its pH factor. A normal skin has a pH factor from 4 to 6. Tests have shown that a skin with a normal pH 4 rises to a pH 7 one minute after washing the face with soap. If cider vinegar is applied to the skin after bathing, the pH factor will remain normal and it is said that no make-up will be needed. Soap made from balsam of Peru makes a soft creamy lather.

Dark circles under the eyes are often the result of lack of sleep and are sure to detract from your looks.

Old eyes become faded and dim. It is said that the following foods will keep the eyes sparkling and lovely, will make the whites of the eyes whiter and by contrast will enhance their colour. These foods are blueberries, tomatoes, avocados, egg plant and sunflower seeds.

Changes in the weather can cause changes in the way the skin behaves. Lack of fresh air and sunshine tends to make the skin sluggish. However, excessive sun exposure can cause wrinkles, dries out the natural moisture of the skin.

Taking pain pills causes a pale, ashen colour of the skin.

Your neck can be a beautiful pedestal for your head or it can have a wrinkled, baggy, lined appearance that betrays your age. Take the same care of the skin on your neck as you do your face.

Women who won't take the time or make the effort to learn about natural means to a youthful looking skin are easily persuaded that hormone creams can do the job.

Harvard dermatologist Dr. H. Blank, upon whose research Revlon bases its claim of its hormone cream, won't commit himself that it works on humans. Many prominent dermatologists say that it definitely will not work.

An extensive study was made by the Council on Pharmacy and Chemistry of the AMA. It is believed that long-continued use of oestrogen face creams may upset normal functioning of the glandular system and may interfere with the natural rhythm of the menstrual period.

Hormones are said to firm sagging skin by water-logging the facial tissues. In this way they stretch the skin and smooth out the wrinkles.

In 1929, an endocrinologist found that if an oestrogen containing cream is rubbed on the shaved back of a castrated mouse, the animal goes into oestrus or heat. In male guinea pigs, he was able to produce growth of the breasts and later milk secretion by rubbing oestrogen hormones into the skin of the back.

The conviction of research scientists is that hormone creams can be absorbed into the skin and cause serious effects such as cancer, since they can create unusual changes in body chemistry.

According to Dr. S. Rothman in his book, *Physiology and Biochemistry of the Skin,* the skin is able to absorb fat-soluble vitamins A and D into the bloodstream. It is his opinion then that the skin would also be able to absorb dangerous poisons used in cosmetics. Dr. Rothman's book mentions hair dyes (anilines, coal-tar dyes), thioglycolic acid used in permanents and unwanted-hair removers, insecticides and oestrogenic hormones.

Users of cosmetics were advised by the Food and Drug Administration to beware of any cosmetics which claim to have mysterious properties.

Don't fall for products that claim to restore a youthful skin or that make promises that appeal to the natural desire of a woman to be beautiful and attractive.

Cosmetics are a poor substitute for your natural heritage. Cosmetic manufacturers sell beauty. They play upon this desire to be attractive. Their advertising pays off handsomely.

There are specific skin-care techniques and natural products that can help you maintain your skin's moisture content.

Cleopatra, who lived in the century preceding the Christian era, was thoroughly versed in the art of using natural cosmetics. Her powders and ointments were crude compared with those arrayed on cosmetic counters, but her formulas were effective aids to beauty.

I find it interesting to experiment with many of these beauty secrets of the ancients.

The following natural oils are all very effective in beauty treatment. Oil of quince, oil of avocado, oil of apricot (kernel), almond oil, sesame oil, wheat-germ oil. The following ingredients are also helpful: Lecithin, lanolin, honey and natural menthol. You may find a secret blend of ingredients.

An anti-wrinkle lotion may be made with half ounce glycerine, half ounce rosewater, half ounce witch hazel and three tablespoonfuls of honey.

Another good anti-wrinkle lotion can be made with tincture of benzoin, glycerine and honey, to which a few drops of cologne may be added. This lotion was used by the ladies of the past.

Massage warm olive oil into the forehead. This is said to overcome wrinkles. For wrinkles you might also try barley water, to which a few drops of oil of balm of Gilead has been added.

If you live where fresh papaya is available, give your face a pick-up and help to give your skin a velvety feeling. Apply a coat of mashed papaya. Leave on ten minutes. Rest during this time with the feet higher than the head. Follow by washing face with warm water. Then splash on cold water. Papaya contains an enzyme which will help to remove the dead outer layers of skin.

Both glycerine and honey are the oldest moisturizers known.

According to an 1870 cosmetic news item, benzoin is a fragrant resin from Sumatra. It has strange qualities. A little powdered benzoin mixed with fat will keep it from becoming rancid.

The Ladies' New Medical Guide, printed in 1901, extols the virtues of benzoin.

A remarkable wash said to have been used by the ladies of the court of Charles IV was made by a tincture of benzoin in water. A small amount of benzoin with glycerine makes a good hand lotion.

For hands that chap easily, dampen common table salt and rub well into hands after having them in water for a time. Rinse in cool water and dry well.

G

A good hand lotion is made with half ounce glycerine, half ounce rosewater and quarter ounce witch hazel. Shake well.

Glycerine is a most useful agent to add to various preparations as a substitute for alcohol as a preservative. One-quarter part of glycerine to three-quarters parts water will preserve drugs as a tincture.

Fill a glass with Epsom salts. Pour in just enough very hot water and melt it. Add twenty drops of glycerine. This is said to be good for the complexion.

A good bleach may be made with one tablespoonful of lemon juice, one tablespoonful of regular peroxide, one teaspoonful of glycerine and one tablespoonful of witch hazel.

An astringent lotion can be made with three-quarters cup rosewater, one-quarter cup witch hazel, one teaspoonful of cider vinegar, one teaspoonful of honey and one teaspoonful of glycerine.

A good lotion is made with one cup rosewater and glycerine, one-quarter cup witch hazel, one teaspoonful of cider vinegar, one teaspoonful of honey and three tablespoonfuls of sesame oil.

Another good lotion is made with tragacanth shavings, glycerine, rain water to make one pint. Heat moderately until it becomes clear. Add water to make up for evaporation.

For sunburn mix glycerine, witch hazel and sunflower seed oil.

A good bath oil can be made with one pint good vegetable oil, a small amount of liquid shampoo. Beat vigorously. Add a few drops of perfume. Keep bottled. Add two tablespoonfuls to a warm bath.

A bag of meadow sweet placed in the bath water makes a good beauty bath.

Place two tablespoonfuls of peppermint leaves in one pint of water. Let it come to a boil—simmer about five minutes- Strain and mix with one pint cider vinegar. Let this stand for two days. When cool add a few drops of perfume. Place one. half cup in a tub of warm water for a relaxing bath.

Another good beauty bath may be made by placing a handful each of rosemary, lavender and comfrey in a muslin bag. Place the bag in hot bath water for a refreshing bath.

Leave an oily complexion cream on the face during a hot bath. The heat aids the treatment for dry skin.

Camomile and stinging nettle tea are fine beauty teas used externally and internally. Yarrow tea, as a wash, is said to make the skin beautiful and velvet-like. Elder flower ointment is said to beautify the complexion.

Both leaves and roots of comfrey have been called the miracle beauty herb. Only recently has comfrey's special skin properties been found. It contains allantoin, an active moisturizing agent. Already scientists have tried to synthesize this element. They have found a way to make allantoin by the crystaline oxidation of uric acid from cows. Which would you prefer to use on your face? Wrinkles and crow's feet, or ageing skin, is said to disappear with continued use of comfrey.

Before sunbathing, reinforce your blood with iron-rich foods and iron-rich herb teas. You will tan more easily and more evenly.

Nail problems are also health problems. For brittle nails, soak them in glycerine. Lack of calcium may be a cause of brittle nails. Keep your nails healthy looking and attractive by careful care.

Proper posture is also necessary to good health and an attractive appearance.

Holy thistle as a wash is said to be a good deoderant.

Beauty is your most valuable asset. Children admire a pretty mother. A little boy, asked to make up a song about his mother on Candid Camera, said she looks like a clown when she puts on her make-up. Your beauty can't show through a mountain of make-up.

Good grooming and good posture belong in beauty culture. Adequate nutrition and sufficient rest and sleep are among the beauty-seeker's best aids.

Try the mirror test. Look deep into your mirror. Be frank about what you see.

CHAPTER XIII

Your Crowning Glory

YOUR hair should be a frame for your face.

A pure bloodstream, nourished with essential food factors, is extremely important if your hair is to retain its natural strength and sheen.

Hair-growth is a series of steps much like a factory assembly line. Failure at any point along the line prevents or reduces your chance of having healthy, luxuriant hair.

Any disease that impairs the vitality of the body has a direct effect upon the hair.

Loss of hair may be caused by sinusitis, nervous diseases, mental disorders, worry, fever, skin diseases and excessive shampooing.

Hair grows approximately at the rate of one inch in six weeks. There is always a falling of hair. As long as the rate of regrowth keeps pace with the loss, it is no cause for alarm.

Along with hair loss, premature greying is a nutritional warning.

Either of the three following supplements is said to be effective in increasing hair growth:

B complex, B-12, inositol, para-amino acid, pyrodoxin (B-6), and cystine.

Calcium-pantothenate, B-12, inositol, para-amino-benzoic acid, and B-6.

B-1, B-2, B-6, B-12, niacin, calcium-pantothenate, and vitamin E.

The foregoing supplements can be very effective. However, all the vitamins, minerals and food factors are essential to good hair health. The diet suggested by nutritional experts for proper hair nourishment is essentially the kind of well-balanced diet everyone needs for good health and freedom from disease.

In a study of 140 women between the ages of 20 and 60 years, all with a hair-loss problem, almost one in five was found to have a slight iron deficiency.

For luxuriant hair one must have sufficient food sulphur in the diet. Never boil sulphur herbs. Sulphur vegetables should be eaten raw.

Riboflavin stimulates normal hair development. Calcium pantothenate helps to restore normal hair colour and regrowth of hair.

Rats deprived of zinc go bald. Wheat-germ contains zinc.

In the case of total inosital deficiency, one can become completely hairless. Inositol is found in brewer's yeast, wheat-germ, carrots, apples, bananas, molasses, tomatoes, straw-berries, lettuce, cantaloupe and dried peas.

There is scientific proof that sex hormones are essential to the formation of hair substances. The hormones dispensed by the glands regulate hair growth.

Hair growth cannot take place if the pituitary gland has lost its power to emit secretions.

In 1932, Dr. B. Norman Bengston, a Chicago physician, experimented on baldness with some success. He used extracts from the pituitary gland.

It has been found that persons with a diseased thyroid gland lose their hair. Iodine is essential to a healthy thyroid. Sea foods and seaweed are rich in iodine. Sarsaparilla is also a good source of iodine.

Greying of hair appears to be related to the adrenal glands. So perhaps stress and strain, through their action on the adrenals, may actully produce grey hair. There have been cases where a person's hair turned white instantly by shock or fright.

The quality and quantity of the hair depends upon the health of the whole glandular system.

At the University of Wisconsin, animals developed all the B-complex deficiency conditions, including greying of hair, when coffee was added to their usual adequate diet.

Deficiency of at least four B vitamins (PABA, biotin, folic acid and pantothenic acid) appear to affect hair colour.

Tests have been made that show that greyness is influenced by the amount of calcium in the body. Lustreless hair generally is indicative of a calcium deficiency. Hair which is dull is also brittle, has a tendency to split, and does not hold a wave or set.

Cysteine increases hair growth and helps to give strength to the hair follicles. There is a scarcity of cysteine in common foods. It is a valuable source of sulphur. Cysteine is an amino acid produced by the digestion of the acid hydrolysis of protein. It may be produced from methionine in some parts of the normal human body.

Wheat-germ oil has been found to stimulate hair growth. One tablespoonful of cod liver oil daily can help the hair achieve a new beauty. When your hair shines, you shine. Lecithin is also known to build hair tissue. Baldness has also been helped by the addition of one teaspoonful of pure inositol daily to a quart of "tiger's milk".

Tightness of scalp is caused by tension. Tight scalp does not allow sufficient fatty tissue beneath skin of scalp. Increase of nervous tension usually increases the amount of dandruff.

Massage in hair care is recommended. Lower the head and massage gently but firmly the neck region towards the area of threatened baldness morning and night. The use of the slant-board is also recommended. When massaging the scalp, just knead, do not rub.

Treatment with synthetic cortiosteroids has caused baldness.

Don't wash the daylights out of your hair. A study at Cornell University found that shampooing creates a loss of calcium, phosphorus, iron and nitrogen from the hair. Eat more foods containing these minerals and help restore these minerals to the hair.

Before shampooing, rub in hot olive oil, then steam head with towels wrung out of very hot water.

Try using egg for shampoo. It was good in grandmother's day and it is good now.

A salon shampoo contains yuccarone, an extract of yucca

plant roots, a natural ingredient used for centuries by south-western American Indians as a hair wash.

Lemon and vinegar rinses are recommended because they restore the normal acidity of an adult's scalp, which is left in an alkaline state immediately after shampooing.

Frequently quacks claim positive cures for baldness and greying hair.

Many of the hair-care articles so attractively advertised are dangerous to use. Women have been known to lose their hair from the use of hair dyes. Loss of hair has also been recorded from use of permanent-wave solutions. Perforation of the eardrum can result if solution gets into the ears.

A report of deafness from using hair spray was given in the *Indiana Times*, January 30, 1960, by science-writer John Troan.

Dr. B. C. Edelston, writing in the British *Lancet* (August 15, 1959), records that synthetic resins found in hair sprays are not metabolized by the body and some of the resins have been found in the liver, spleen, and lungs. Many of these resins are cancer causing.

Long before the days of beauty salons, women had their own home-made hair treatments. Among these are certain herbs that nourish and brighten the hair. Then why turn to quackery when herb teas are really an effective aid to hair health?

Jaborandi pilocarpus is highly recommended for hair growth.

The leaves and bark of the willow tree are said to rid the hair of dandruff.

An ounce of rosemary, steeped in one pint of boiling water, makes the best hair wash or rinse known. Some commercial shampoos contain rosemary.

A handful of stinging nettle, boiled in one quart of water (or use cider vinegar and water), makes an excellent hair tonic. It also darkens grey hair.

Marigold flowers were used in the past for tinting blond hair.

Women of past years used sage and camomile rinses. Today you can still find these rinses in modern salons, either in their natural form or disguised under a fancy name or label.

A tea of camomile flowers will bring out the lustre and highlights of blond hair. Boil three tablespoonfuls of the dried flowers in one pint of water for twenty minutes.

A sage rinse is used to darken gery hair. It is not a dye. It is made by boiling one ounce of sage leaves in one quart of water for twenty minutes or more. The longer it is allowed to boil the darker will be the colour rinse.

Rub either of these rinses well into the scalp. They will wash out with the next shampoo. Remove thoroughly, however, before the next permanent.

Twigs of wild cherry have also been used effectively to make a good hair tonic.

Simmer one-half gallon cider vinegar in oven to which the following has been added: Rosemary leaves, peach tree leaves, camomile flowers, jaborandi leaves and southernwood ashes. This is said to grow hair.

A good hair oil is made with rosemary (oil and leaves), egg yolk, soapwort, papaya leaves, stinging nettle, yarrow, sunflower seed oil and glycerine.

An old recipe for baldness was made by steeping four ounces of wild indigo for about a week or ten days in one pint of alcohol and one pint of water. Apply morning and evening with a sponge or soft brush.

An old recipe for greying hair is made by distilling two pounds of honey, one handful rosemary leaves and twelve handfuls of grape tendrils. Infuse in one gallon of water.

The Indiana Botanic Gardens of Hammond, Indiana, had the following recipe in their almanac:

2	boxes	haar wurzel
1	box	jaborandi leaves
½	„	sage leaves
1	„	camomile flowers
1	„	peach tree leaves

Place the above in a gallon jar. Add one quart cider vinegar and two quarts of water. Let stand ten days, then strain. Apply to scalp morning and night. Allow to dry without rinsing. They claim it is a good dandruff remover if used warm as a hair wash in place of shampooing the hair. The Indiana Botanic Gardens also has this formula already prepared. Incidentally, I buy all my herbs from this company. I find their herbs are clean and good.

To darken the hair, place two ounces green tea and two ounces sage leaves in three quarts of boiling water. Cover and let simmer until liquid has been reduced to one quart. Allow this to stand twenty-four hours. Strain and bottle.

Culpepper and Banckc both wrote, "Ashes of Southernwood mixed with oil restoreth where a man lacketh hair".

Plantain and shepherd's purse are also recommended to improve the texture and sheen of the hair.

Any of the following herbs are said to nourish and brighten the hair: Peppergrass, marshmallow leaves and mullein leaves.

Thousands of dollars are spent yearly by women at the numerous modern beauty salons. Most of this money is spent for permanents and hair sets.

A hair shaft is flat and porous. As it absorbs moisture, it becomes shorter and curls up.

Hair soaked in an alkaline solution and heated is said to curl.

One of the ingredients used in commercial permanents is thioglycolate, which is also used in the manufacture of unwanted-hair removers.

Thio is a combining form denoting the presence of sulphur. Glycol is found in unripe grapes.

Among the sulphur herbs are mullein, eyebright, and stinging nettle.

Sodium is the most important alkaline element.

Sodium herbs are shepherd's purse, nettle and fennel seed.

A fine hair-curling solution is made with one part of gum arabic and four parts of rosewater, to which a few drops of sesame oil, wheat-germ oil, a very small amount of pure lanolin and one tablespoonful of glycerine are added.

Apple pectin has also been used.

Another good hair-curling solution is made by mixing half dram gum tragacanth, half pint water, three ounces glycerine and ten drops rose compound oil. Cover and let stand twenty-four hours. Strain and bottle.

Warm water is better than hot for shampoos.

Strained lemon juice as a final rinse leaves hair clean and lustrous. Add juice to the last rinse. One tablespoonful of vinegar is also good in the final rinse. Both help restore the natural pH factor of the scalp after shampooing.

Always wash combs and brushes at time of every shampoo. Cleanliness is the best protection against dandruff and falling hair. Wash combs and brushes in warm water to which one tablespoonful of ammonia has been added.

Blame has been placed for hair loss in women on injury by stiff hairbrushes and the continuous pull produced by pony-tail hair styles and by rolling curlers too tight.

The late Helena Rubenstein said, "You have to live with your hair a long, long time, so treat it with respect".

Take stock of your hair needs. Pamper your hair back to health, beauty and manageability. Preserve it with natural means.

CHAPTER XIV

The Art of Perfumery

PERFUMERY is an interesting sideline to beauty culture.

To make an old-fashioned violet perfume, place twelve drops of oil of rhodium on a piece of loaf sugar and reduce to a fine powder. Mix thoroughly with three pounds of orris root (powdered). This will resemble violet perfume. Add more oil and you will have a rose perfume.

Place rose petals in water. Add a few drops of vitriolic acid. Soon the water will take on the colour and fragrance of roses.

Place two pounds of rose petals on a cloth tied around the edge of a pan filled with hot water. Keep the water hot. Place a dish of cold water upon the petals. Change the water on top as soon as it gets warm. By this method of distillation, which is inexpensive, quite a large quantity of the essential oil of roses is extracted.

Sweet basil is a sweet-smelling herb that is used in perfumery.

Another method of making perfume which was used in the past is as follows. Put rose petals (or any fragrant flowers) in a can. Press full. Put in all the glycerine that the can will hold. Cover tightly. In three or four weeks the perfume will be extracted.

A good cologne is said to be made by mixing twelve ounces of rosemary leaves, one ounce fresh lemon peel, one ounce fresh orange peel, one ounce dried mint leaves, one ounce lemon balm, one pint strong rosewater and one pint alcohol. Let stand eight or ten days.

Sachet bags were quite popular in colonial days. They make original gifts. There are several methods of making sachet bags.

Mix one ounce of cloves, caraway seeds, nutmeg, mace, cinnamon and tonquin beans (all powdered). Add as much

Florentine orris root (powdered) as will equal the other ingredients put together. Place in fancy little bags.

Ground rose petals, two ounces tonquin beans and one ounce vanilla beans. Reduce to powder and mix. Sift dry ingredients and add two drops of oil of almonds. This makes a good sachet.

For a lavender fragrance, take half pound powdered lavender flowers, quarter pound powdered gum benzoin and one and a quarter ounces of oil of lavender.

Ground fennel seed is also used in sachet bags.

Also mix well one pound orris root and one pound acacia flowers for a good sachet.

Grind one ounce each of coriander seeds, wild ginger root, and lavender flowers, one-half ounces each of deer's tongue and sweet flag root.

Mix and sift six pounds orris root, bergamot four ounces, four onces acacia flowers and one-quarter ounces cloves.

Mix well one ounce lavender flowers, one-half ounce each of orris root and rosemary leaves and five drops oil of rose.

Sandalwood is excellent as an incense or used in sachets.

Other botanicals used in perfumery, sachets and *pot-pourri* are calamus root, costmary leaves, lemon verbena, rose buds, sandalwood and khus-khus (also called vetivert).

Scented cakes will perfume your wardrobe and also kill moths. Melt one ounce paraffin. Add ten grains of heliotropin. Then add five drops of oil of bergamot and two drops of oil of cloves. When cool cut in cakes. Wrap in foil until ready for use.

Pot-pourri or rose jars make excellent gifts. There are different ways to make *pot-pourri*. One way is to gather rose petals each day and partially dry them in the sun. When they are fairly dry, put them in an attractive container. To every two ounces of dried petals add one ounce of powdered orris root and a sprinkling of salt or a few drops of glycerine. Let this stand for about two weeks, stirring often until it is perfectly dry. Then add one-quarter ounce each of allspice and cinnamon and one-eighth ounce of cloves and one ounce of dried lavender. Dried borage flowers may be added, not for fragrance, but they retain a lovely blue colour when dried and will add to the attractiveness of your jar. One tonka bean may be added to increase the fragrance. The leaves must be thoroughly dry or the *pot-pourri* will mould. When well made this *pot-pourri* should last for years. If it loses its perfume, stir well. Each year you may add dried rose petals, lavender and spices and salt to freshen up the jar. This is said to remain fragrant in open jars for two years and much longer in closed containers.

CHAPTER XV

Herbal Beverages

HERBAL beverages can be tasty thirst quenchers. A combination of herbs as a beverage is an excellent source of all the elements needed for perfect metabolic balance.

Select two or three or as many as you wish, from the following: Alfalfa, red clover blossoms, stinging nettle, violet leaves and flowers, camomile flowers, spearmint, peppermint, rosemary, sage, balm (melissa officinalis), garden rue, borage, sarsaparilla, sassafras and elder flowers. These are my choice of beverage herbs.

The Ojibwe Indians made a cooling drink of sumac berries in summer and made it hot in winter.

Sweet-scented golden rod is an agreeable substitute for tea. A good tea can also be made with the leaves of the persimmon tree.

Barley water forms a particularly bland and demulcent drink. With honey or brown sugar and lemon juice added, it makes a delicious beverage. Powdered rosehips added to this drink, in place of the lemon juice, is also good. Rosehips makes a tasty addition to any herbal beverage.

Grape juice, cranberry juice, apple juice, elderberry juice, pineapple juice and other wild and tame juices make a delicious drink singly or in combinations.

Try these beverages on your children, they will go for them in a big way and they are harmless.

CHAPTER XVI

Help for the Smoker

THERE are many who want to stop smoking. To do so can be very trying. As a result of cigarette smoking, the nervous system is definitely affected. For this reason it is so difficult to break the habit.

There are tablets on the market to help stop this vicious habit but, here again, I would refrain from using anything of a chemical nature when from the herbal kingdom there are herbs that one can rely on as being harmless and which can give hope to those who need help to overcome this habit.

The first step that I would suggest is to take a mild sedative. Here is where we can turn with confidence to herbs for help. Tranquillizers and other chemical nerve medicines can only do harm, but an herbal calmative is safe. A combination of lady-slipper, scullcap, valerian, catnip and peppermint is the best and safest sedative one can take. It acts directly on the whole nervous system to calm it and to strengthen it.

Another thing the individual who tries to stop smoking must contend with is a ferocious appetite. He is always hungry. Here is where a good nourishing diet is especially important. A diet containing all of the necessary food elements is so much needed here.

Another suggestion is to exercise freely in the open air. Climbing a hill is especially good exercise if the heart can take it.

Life is a process of oxidation. Air must enter the body continually to carry on this process. Outdoor exercising offers enough oxygen for the lungs to carry on their important work and to aid in the cleansing and healing of every part of the body, which is so important when trying to discontinue smoking. When the air we breathe is polluted, the lungs are certain to be harmed. The mucous membrane of the lungs is injured and the lungs are definitely weakened.

Since cigarette smoking is a habit, help must be given along that line. It is claimed that substituting something to put into the mouth is a help. Sucking on candy or chewing gum is suggested. Let the candy be made with honey. Honey alone, a teaspoonful taken now and then when the craving becomes unbearable, has helped some.

There are herbs listed as aids to help curb the smoking habit. Besides those herbs I suggested as a calmative, tea made from magnolia leaves, angelica root and sassafras is said to be effective. Chewing a mixture of liquorice root and "life everlasting" is also said to be helpful. These are all harmless.

I would suggest making a strong tea of the magnolia, angelica and sassafras. Strain and add enough honey to make honey drops to be sucked when the craving comes on.

By resorting to pipe smoking, one can cut down on the nicotene content by adding botanicals to the tobacco as the Indians did. The more botanics added, the less nicotine will be in the smoke.

The crushed berries of allspice are used in the West Indies for their spicy aroma.

A main ingredient in one good herbal smoke mixture is coltsfoot together with eyebright, rosemary, thyme and camomile.

"Life everlasting" is a popular pipe smoke among European peasants.

Mullein and corn silk were used by the American Indians, alone or with tobacco. The Indians also smoked sassafras bark.

Gentian makes a good substitute for tobacco. Sweet clover has also been used as a smoke.

In the *Historical Dictionary*, printed in 1813, is an account of the use of the berries of sumach (Rhus glabra) as a substitute for tobacco. It is said to be an antidote for the smoke habit. The berries should be gathered in November. Expose for a time in the open air, then dry in a slow oven. Then spread them out for twenty-two hours, when it will be ready for use. The

Western American Indians made a preparation of equal parts of the roots and leaves of sumach, which they smoked under the name of Kinikah.

The fresh inner bark of the white poplar may be chewed, or mix the powdered bark with powdered sugar and extract of liquorice and compress into small tablets, five grains of the bark each. When a desire to smoke comes on, dissolve one in the mouth.

Colombo root is said to be a good substitute for tobacco. It is claimed to stop the craving.

Comfrey is also said to be a tobacco substitute. It is supposed to make quite an enjoyable smoke and has a healing effect on the lungs.

One smoker lost all desire to smoke by eating copious amounts of apples and other fresh fruits.

When a smoker craves a smoke, encourage him to drink a glass of some liquid, water, fruit juice, vegetable juice or milk. Also a teaspoonful of honey will help to get over the craving.

If, at the close of meals, fruits such as oranges, grapefruit, peaches or apples are eaten, it will help to lessen the desire for that after dinner smoke. It is also advised to drink water and buttermilk freely.

In the case of overcoming the smoking habit, there is nothing that will equal the old saying, "Where there is a will, there is a way." A strong will is especially important to overcome this vicious habit.

For the throat irritation due to smoking, mix equal parts of hyssop, horchound, coltsfoot and marshmallow root. Make a tea with three or four teaspoons to a tea pot. Drink one cupful as desired. A syrup made with this tea and honey is perhaps better.

Vicious greed that promotes advertising to make one feel that it is smart to smoke is the aim of cigarette manufacturers. They have made use of the knowledge that children are great imitators by promoting the making of candy cigarettes with names so similar to the real brands that children might be impressed by cigarette advertising. A powder is puffed from these candy cigarettes to resemble smoke.

You can see how great is our responsibility to our boys and girls.

H

CHAPTER XVII

Herbs and their Properties

Alfalfa: Buffalo herb, lucerne

Alfalfa is one of the richest land-grown sources of sub-nutritional trace food minerals. The deep feeder roots go down deep into the soil, fifty feet and more, to bring those much needed trace minerals. Most food plants are shallow surface feeders. Alfalfa is considered one of the best sources of iron, magnesium, phosphorus, sulphur, sodium, potassium, chlorine and silicon. It is particularly rich in plant calcium. It is one of the best plant sources of vitamin K, which is so essential to the clotting of blood. Alfalfa also contains eight known enzymes, so necessary to make foods assimilable by the body. In his book, *Medicinal Value of Natural Foods*, Dr. W. H. Graves, D.C., lists alfalfa as indicated in cases of diabetes, TB, rheumatism, Bright's Disease, toxaemia, jaundice, neuralgia, insomnia, nervousness, syphilis, constipation, lumbago, hardening of the arteries, dropsy, prostatitis, anaemia, skin eruptions and poor complexion. It is also listed as a good blood builder, good for teeth and bones and for inflamed bladder. It is a splendid milk producer for nursing mothers. It greatly aids in the elimination of various drug poisons from the body. *Government Bulletin No. 247* says: "The results show that 90% of the potassium, 85% of the magnesium, 75% of the phosphorus, 50% of the nitrogen and 40% of the calcium contained in the dried alfalfa plant are soluble in water."

Aloes: Aloes Vera, Aloe Socotrina

PART USED: Leaves

Cathartic, stomachic, aromatic, emmenagogue

One of the best herbs to clean out the colon, promote menstruation when suppressed. Will expel worms after several doses. Start with small dose when used as a cathartic. Cleans morbid matter from the stomach, liver, kidneys, spleen and bladder. Excellent for burns, radiation burns, cuts and bruises. For singers and speakers, clears throat. Merely cut off one-quarter inch of one leaf and chew and keep in the mouth a few minutes and finally swallow.

Althea: Althea Officinalis, Mallow Family, Marshmallow
PART USED: Root
Emollient, demulcent, pain-soothing
As a douche for irritation of the vagina. Bathing inflamed eyes. In making poultices. Irritative diarrhoea or dysentery. Dried root may be chewed and the saliva swallowed for soothing inflamed bladder or kidneys and all mucous membranes.

Angelica: Angelica Atropurpurea, Archangel
PART USED: Root and seed
Stimulant, aromatic, carminative, diaphoretic, expectorant, diuretic, emmenagogue
A good tonic. For stomach trouble, heartburn, gas, colic, colds and fever. Tea dropped into the eye helps dimness of sight. Dropped into the ears, helps deafness. Strengthens the heart. Effective in epidemics. In case of poisons, take in morning, fasting if possible. Powdered root is reputed to cause disgust for all spirituous liquors.

Anise: Pimpinella anisum
PART USED: Seed
Stimulant and carminative
Used for colic in infants, to remove nausea, prevent fermentation of gas in stomach and bowels. Aids digestion. Overcomes disturbances caused by overeating.

Annatto: Achiote
PART USED: Seed
Contains more vitamin A and D than cod-liver oil.

Arnica: Arnica Montana, Leopard's Bane
PART USED: Flowers
Emetic and Cathartic
Used preferably externally in liniments for bruises, strains, sprains, pain, muscular rheumatism.

Asparagus: Asparagus officinale
PART USED: The herb
Diuretic

Good as a heart sedative and for kidney and bladder stones and dropsy.

Balm of Gilead: Populus Balsamifera or Candicans
PART USED: Buds
Stimulant, expectorant

The resinous substance is not acted upon by water alone. An infusion cannot be made. Boiled in oil makes an excellent ointment or salve. Valuable in colds, lung, kidney and urinary difficulties.

Basil (sweet): Ocium basilicum, Ocymum
PART USED: Leaves
Stimulant, condiment, nervine, aromatic

Tea taken hot is good in suppressed menstruation. Allays excessive vomiting. Effective when applied to snake bites and insect stings. Expels afterbirth.

Black Cohosh: Cimicifuga racemosa
PART USED: Root
Relaxant, expectorant, slightly narcotic sedative, antispasmodic, nervine

Exerts a marked influence over the nervous system. For epilepsy, convulsions, acute rheumatism, sciatica, St. Vitus Dance, neuralgia, spinal meningitis, snake-bite poisoning, delirium tremens. Brings on menstrual flow retarded by cold or exposure. Relieves cramp in menstrual period. Wonderful remedy for high blood pressure and whooping cough.

Black Haw: Viburnum prunifolium
PART USED: Bark of root
Diuretic, tonic, antispasmodic, nervine, astringent

Counteracts threatened abortion. Relieves after pains. Good for ovarian irritation, asthma, hysteria. A valuable ingredient of female tonics.

Blue Cohosh: Caulophyllum thalictroides
PART USED: Root
Emmenagogue, parturient, antispasmodic

Valuable remedy in epilepsy, uterine disorders, leucorrhoea, dropsy, cramp, colic, hysteria, diabetes, high blood pressure. Helps to alkalinize blood and urine. Makes childbirth easy. An infusion taken for a week or two preceding confinement renders delivery comparatively rapid and painless.

Blue Flag: Iris versicolour
PART USED: The rhizome
Alterative, cathartic, sialogogue, vermifuge, diuretic.
Has a special affinity for the thyroid gland.

Boneset: Eupatorium perfoliatium
PART USED: Tops and leaves
Relaxant, sudorific, antiseptic, stimulant, diuretic
Infusion valuable in intermittent and typhoid fevers, general debility, epidemic influenza. A large dose of warm infusion is emetic. Produces perspiration, promotes all secretions. Taken cold it is laxative and tonic. Breaks up colds. Is extremely bitter.

Borage: Borago officinalis
PART USED: The herb
Pectoral, cordial, aperient
Expels poisons. Rich in potassium and calcium. Comforts the heart when saddened with much grief. All the glandular system is gradually influenced by the singular action of borage. Used to defend the heart in contagious or eruptive fevers. Seeds and leaves are said to increase mother's milk. Good to bathe sore eyes. Valuable in hepatitis.

Buchu: Barosma crenata
PART USED: Leaves
Aromatic, stimulant, diuretic, diaphoretic
Inflammation of the bladder, irritation of the membrane of the urethra, incontinence of urine.

Burdock: Arctium lappa, Lappa minor
PART USED: Root
Diuretic, depilatory, alterative
One of the best blood purifiers. Cleanses and eliminates

impurities from the blood very rapidly. Will clear all skin diseases, boils and carbuncles. Made into a salve for skin eruptions, burns, wounds and haemorrhoids. Increases flow of urine. An especially good diuretic for children. Also good for sciatica, leprosy. Excellent to reduce weight. Place green root, mashed fine, in water, stir well, let stand a half day. Drink freely. Dried root also used. Use only one-year-old roots. Dig in spring or autumn. Burdock-leaf poultice allays inflammation and pain. Bruise leaves for bruises and sprains. Gives immediate relief.

Camomile: Anthemis nobilis
PART USED: Flowers
Tonic

Produces perspiration. Promotes menstrual flow. Will soften skin. Good during convalescence. For quinsy, boil in water and inhale steam. Strengthens and gives tone to the stomach. Expels gas. Aids digestion. Prevents fermentation in the stomach. Good n female troubles, colic in infants, intermittent fever and typhoid. Especially good for babies while teething. A poultice of camomile will often prevent gangrene and remove it when present. Also good in pulmonary complaints.

Caraway: Carum carui
PART USED: Seed
Carminative, stimulant, diuretic, stomachic

Colic in infants. Strengthens and gives tone to the stomach. Good for female troubles (side ache). Powdered seeds made into a poultice will remove black and blue spots of bruises. The roots of caraway may be eaten as parsnips.

Cascara Sagrada: Rhamnus purschiana, Sacred Bark
Purgative, tonic, febrifuge

Old Indian remedy for constipation. Increases secretions of stomach, liver and pancreas. Excellent for children for constipation. A good intestinal tonic. Best results when combined with other purgative herbs. Improves with age. Not habit forming.

Catnip: Nepeta cataria, Nip
PART USED: The whole herb

Carminative, stimulant, tonic, diaphoretic, antispasmodic, aphrodisiac

Excellent for its quieting effect on the nervous system. Use as an enema for children, especially in convulsions. Very useful in pain of any kind, for spasms, insanity, fevers, colic, hysteria, amenorrhoea, emmenagogue, nervous headache. An enema of catnip will cause urination when it has stopped. Catnip, sweet balm, marshmallow and sweet weed (liquorice) make an excellent baby remedy, nervous irritability, colds and hoarseness. Used hot in connection with a hot foot-bath is very beneficial for colds.

Cayenne: Capsicum annuum

PART USED: Fruit

Stimulant, antiseptic

One of the strongest and purest stimulants known. The key to success in medicine is stimulation. Since stimulation is so important in most every form of disease, it is a valuable adjunct to other medicines. May be used in all cases of debility, indigestion, costiveness, chills, heart failure. Cayenne acts mainly upon the circulation. Its influence is immediate on the heart. Gives tone to the circulation. A good addition to cathartics to prevent griping. In constipation, cayenne stimulates the peristaltic motion of the bowels. For this purpose give daily in small doses. Cayenne is good for coughs, colds, quinsy, diphtheria, scarlet fever, and sore throat. For asthma combine cayenne with lobelia. For toothache, clean out cavity, place cotton saturated with oil of capsicum into cavity. Beneficial effect should last for months. One-half teaspoonful of cayenne in hot foot-bath for apoplexy. If taken with meals will help digestion. For pleurisy, three No. 4 capsules every hour should relieve pain. Wonderful for lock-jaw, combined with lobelia. Good in cases of spring fever, lethargy, yellow fever and all other fevers. Also for haemorrhages of the lungs. In quinsy and diphtheria, apply tincture on neck. Then place a piece of flannel around neck. Infusion taken internally along with external application. Cayenne arouses all the secreting organs. Will ultimately reach every organ of the body. It is a most persistent heart stimulant. Will heal a sore ulcerated stomach. Give frequently and in small doses.

Celery: Apium graveolens
PART USED: Root and seed
Diuretic, stimulant, aromatic
Used in incontinence of the urine, dropsy, liver troubles. Produces perspiration. A splendid tonic. Good for nervousness, neuralgia and rheumatism.

Chestnut: Castania
PART USED: Leaves
Antispasmodic
Soothing to mucous membranes and the nervous system. A specific for whooping cough (combined with blue cohosh and lobelia). Good for other coughs too. For protracted cases of hiccoughs.

Chickweed: Stellaria Media, Starwort, Satin Flower, Stitchwort
PART USED: Leaves
Alterative, demulcent, refrigerant, mucilaginous, pectoral, resolvent, discutient
Chickweed may be used fresh, dried or powdered in poultices, fomentations or salves. Excellent in bronchitis, pleurisy, coughs, colds, hoarseness, rheumatism, inflammation of the bowels and stomach. Heals and soothes anything it comes in contact with. It is one of the best remedies for external application to skin diseases, boils, burns, sore eyes, tumours, erysipelas, haemorrhoids and sore throat. Take a chickweed bath for skin diseases. For blood poisoning take internally as well as application of a chickweed poultice. Chickweed, especially eaten fresh, is an excellent as well as harmless treatment for obesity.

Chicory: Cichorium endiva
PART USED: Root
Tonic, laxative, diuretic
Disorders of kidneys, liver, stomach and spleen. For jaundice. Settles upset stomach. Tones up system. Mix chicory with coffee.

Cleavers: Galium aparine
PART USED: Whole herb
Refrigerant, diuretic, aperient, alterative, tonic

Makes an excellent wash for the face to clear the complexion. A good blood cleanser. Excellent in all cases of fever, scarlet fever, measles, eczema. Excellent in jaundice, bladder stones and dropsy. Stops bleeding of wounds. Good for old sores. Cooked in broth, it is a good reducing aid.

Colombo: Cocculus palmatus
PART USED: Root
Anti-emetic, tonic, febrifuge

One of the best and purest tonics to strengthen and tone up the entire system. Useful in fevers. Excellent to allay vomiting in pregnancy; colon trouble, even of long standing; chronic diarrhoea, cholera. Taken after overeating, is a good stomach remedy. Improves appetite. A bitter tonic.

Coltsfoot: Tussilago farfara
PART USED: Root and leaves
Emollient, demulcent, expectorant, pectoral, diaphoretic, tonic

Excellent remedy for sinusitis, and all lung troubles. Very soothing to mucous membranes. Loosens phlegm in coughs, asthma, bronchitis, whooping cough, spasmodic cough, taken as a cough syrup. Also good for shortness of breath, ague and fevers.

Comfrey: Symphytum officinale
PART USED: Root and leaves
Demulcent, astringent, pectoral, vulnerary, mucilaginous, styptic, nutritive

Powerful remedy in coughs, tickling coughs, sinusitis, lung trouble, asthma, ulceration of kidneys, stomach or bowels. For bloody urine. Fomentations wrung out of strong tea for bruises, sprains and fractures. Will relieve pain. Poultice of fresh leaves excellent for ruptures, fresh wounds, burns, gangrene and moist ulcers. Poultice also gives relief to painful joints. Also good to make salve.

Coriander: Coriandrum satium
PART USED: Seed
Aromatic, stomachic, cordial, pungent, carminative
   Good stomach tonic. Strengthening to heart. Allays griping caused by other laxatives. Expels gas from bowels. Used in confections.

Corn Silk: Stigmata Maidis, Zea Mays
Demulcent, diuretic
   For irritable condition of urinary organs. Excellent for bed-wetting (enuresis) when combined with agrimony. One of the best remedies for kidney, bladder and prostate trouble.

Creeping Jenny: European bindweed
   Bleeding stopped instantly when the roots touch the wound.

Dandelion: Taraxicum dens-leonis
PART USED: Leaves and root
Hepatic, aperient, diuretic, depurative, tonic, stomachic
   Purifies blood. Destroys acids in blood. Excellent for anae-mia. Root is used to increase flow of urine. Is slightly laxative. Good for jaundice, eczema, kidney trouble, dropsy, inflam-mation of bowels and fever. Has a beneficial effect on female organs. Increases activity of liver, pancreas and spleen. Good in enlargement of liver and spleen. An excellent sub-stitute for coffee. A slow tonic. Good when combined with peach leaves. Also good for nervous debility. Root combined with cayenne and lobelia makes a good tonic. Also good for diseases of the skin and for uterine obstructions. Root must be boiled.

Dill: Anethum graveolens
PART USED: Seed
Stomachic, aromatic, stimulant, carminative, diaphoretic
   Very quieting to the nerves. Stops hiccoughs. Strengthening to brain. Expels gas.

Elecampane: Inula helenium
PART USED: Root
Diaphoretic, diuretic, expectorant, aromatic, stimulant, sto-machic, astringent, tonic
   Useful in whooping cough. Strengthens, cleanses and tones

up pulmonary and gastric membranes. For retention of urine. Delayed menstruation. Also for kidney and bladder stones. Clears and strengthens sight. Good in weakness of digestive organs. For torpor of liver. A stimulating expectorant. A good formula consists of elecampane, spikenard (one ounce each) and four ounces wild cherry bark. Also elecampane and comfrey.

Elderberry: Sambucus
PART USED: Flowers, berries and root
Diaphoretic, gently stimulant, diuretic, alterative, aperient

Flowers in infusion-hepatic derangements of children, erysipelas. Expressed juice of the berries will purge. Juice will also promote all fluid secretions. Much used in dropsy. Blossoms beaten up with lard make a good ointment in burns, scalds. Inner bark has been used by taking from branches one or two years old and scraping off the grey outer bark. I have used the blossoms together with peppermint leaves, the tea sweetened with a little honey, for colds with exceptional results. I have given small amounts to very small children who were close to having pneumonia and overnight they were much improved. I have also simmered the blossoms in vegetable oil and applied it warm to caked breasts with fine results. When one of our boys was eight months old, he was severely burned about the face, chest and one arm. Everyone who saw him was certain he would be scarred for life. That night I had a dream. I was shown how to make an ointment to apply to his burns. Elderberry blossom was one of the ingredients I was shown to use. Today he has no trace of a scar. The berries also have therapeutic virtues. They have been found to contain as much if not more vitamin C than orange juice. An ointment can be made with the blossoms to beautify the complexion.

Eyebright: Euphrasia officinale
PART USED: Leaves
Tonic astringent

Coughs, hoarseness, headache, earache, sinusitis, dimness of sight (to be used internally as well as an eye wash). Restores sight decayed through age. Said to restore sight to those who were blind a long time. Helps the memory.

Fennel: Foeniculum officinale
PART USED: Seeds and leaves
Stomachic, carminative, pectoral, diuretic, diaphoretic, aromatic

Tea makes an excellent eyewash. Relieves gas, helps acid stomach, good for cramp and for colic in infants. Eliminates poisons. Excellent for obesity. Increases menstrual flow. Increases flow of urine. Fennel boiled with barley is good for nursing mothers, increases milk. Stops hiccoughs.

Fenugreek: Trigonella foenum graecum
PARTS USED: Seed
Mucilaginous, farinaceous

Poultice excellent for wounds. Tea is an excellent gargle for sore throat. Seed boiled in soy milk or nut milk is very nourishing. Excellent in fevers. Cooling to bowels. Lubricates the intestines. Be careful though, it is said to make people plump.

Fleabane: Erigeron caradense
PART USED: The whole plant
Styptic, astringent, diuretic, tonic

Excellent for summer complaint, especially for children when all other remedies fail. Colon trouble. Bladder trouble, scalding urine, haemorrhages from bowels and uterus. Use in an enema.

Gentian: Gentiana lutea
PART USED: Root
Stomachic, tonic, anthemintic, antibilious

Powerful and effective and reliable tonic. Purifies blood. Good for liver complaints. Excellent in spleen affections. Improves appetite. Strengthens digestive organs. Increases circulation. Invigorates entire system. Useful in fevers, colds. Expels worms. Excellent in suppressed menstruation. For scanty urine. Remedy against intermittent fever in malarial countries. Acts like quinine. Allays poisons from mad-dog bites, insect and snake bites. For chills, hourly doses with a little cayenne added.

Ginseng: Panax quinquefolia
PART USED: Root
Demulcent, stomachic, slightly stimulant
Promotes appetite. Useful in digestive disturbances. For colds, chest troubles and coughs. Will produce perspiration when taken hot. Good for constipation, inflammation of urinary tract. The Chinese take ginseng as a precautionary measure against diseases of every kind.

Golden seal: Hydrastis canadensis
PART USED: Root
Laxative, tonic, alterative, detergent, opthalmicum, antiperiodic, aperient, diuretic, antiseptic, deobstruent
One of the best remedies in the whole herbal kingdom. Excellent for colds, 'flu, stomach and liver trouble. Exerts a good influence on all mucous membranes. Excellent for open sores, eczema, ringworm, erysipelas, any skin disease. In small doses, will allay nausea during pregnancy. Equalizes circulation. Combined with skullcap and cayenne, strengthens the heart. Combined with myrrh for ulcerated stomach. Especially good for enlarged tonsils. Will improve appetite and aid digestion. Combined with skullcap and hops for a very fine tonic for spinal nerves. Very good in spinal meningitis. Useful in all skin eruptions. scarlet fever and smallpox. For pyorrhoea, dip toothbrush in the powder and brush teeth. Useful in typhoid fever, leucorrhoea. Combined with peach leaves, queen of the meadow, cleavers and cornsilk, it is good for Bright's disease and diabetes. Golden seal is good to bathe the eyes. Chronic catarrh of the stomach. Good for malarial poisoning or enlarged spleen. For diarrhoea, combine golden seal with raspberries. Sustains circulation of the blood. Golden seal and cayenne taken to prevent pain in stomach after eating. Gargle with tea for diphtheria. A powerful tonic. Children take smaller doses.

Gotu Kola: Hydrocotyle asiatica
PART USED: Leaves
Leaves have a marked energizing effect on the cells of the brain and are said to preserve the brain indefinitely. It is not a

stimulant, but a brain food. Powdered leaves in small doses in cow's milk for mental weakness and memory improvement. A few leaves eaten raw are said to strengthen and revitalize worn out bodies and brains to a remarkable degree. Will prevent brain fag and nervous breakdown. Also a leprosy cure and good for hepatitis.

Hops: Humulus Lupulus
PART USED: Cones
Febrifuge, tonic, nervine, diuretic, anodyne, hypnotic, anthelmintic, sedative

Excellent nervine, sleeplessness. Cough syrup. Hot fomentation to face for neuralgia. Poultice for abscesses. Good for delirium tremens, toothache. Tones up liver. Increases flow of urine. Increases flow of bile. For diseases in throat and chest. Hot poultices effective for boils, tumours and pain and old ulcers. Used for after-pains. Honey combined with hops and a little lobelia is excellent for bronchitis. Added to ordinary gargles.

Horehound: Marrubium vulgare
PART USED: Whole plant
Pectoral, aromatic, diaphoretic, tonic, expectorant, diuretic, hepatic, stimulant

Will produce profuse perspiration when taken hot. In large doses it is laxative. Good for jaundice, asthma, hysteria. Will expel worms. Useful in coughs, sore throat. When menstruation stops abnormally, will bring about flow again. Especially good for croup. Will expel afterbirth. Eliminates poisons. Honey and horehound are said to clear the vision.

Horsemint: Monarda Punctata
PART USED: Leaves and tops
Aromatic, pungent, bitter, carminative, stimulant, nervine, diuretic, diaphoretic, antiseptic

New drug from Monarda Punctata for athlete's foot, psoriasis, ringworm and impetigo.

Hyssop: Hyssopus officinalis
PART USED: Whole plant

Aromatic, sudorific, pectoral, expectorant, febrifuge, anthelmintic, aperient, stimulant, carminative, tonic.

An old Bible remedy. Increases circulation, Reduces blood pressure. Kills body lice and hair lice. Expels worms. Used in jaundice, dropsy, for the spleen. Removes discolouration of bruises. Excellent for fevers and for wash for the eyes. Used in quinsy and sore throat, asthma and coughs, fevers and spasms of infants. Cold infusion is a good tonic and stimulant.

Juniper: Juniperus communis
PART USED: Bark and berries
Diuretic, gently stimulant
Effective for kidney, urinary and bladder trouble. Excellent as a spray for fumigation. Preventive of disease. Berries can be chewed, or a strong tea used as a gargle when exposed to contagious diseases; a good immunizer. Too large doses may cause irritation in the urinary passage. A counter-poison. Good in dropsy and gravel. Assures a safe, speedy delivery. Strengthens the brain, memory and optic nerve. Used in leprosy and ague. Combine with peach leaves and a little marshmallow for good results.

Lady Slipper: Cypripedium Pubescens
PART USED: Root. Should be gathered in August or September.
Tonic, stimulant, diaphoretic, antispasmodic
Excellent for hysteria, nervous irritability, nervous headache.

Liquorice: Glycirrhiza glabra
PART USED: Root
Demulcent, expectorant, laxative
Suitable for coughs. Best combined with black cohosh and wild cherry. Maidenhair and figs combined with liquorice is also a good combination. A pleasant drink may be made with flaxseed, ginger, lemon, honey or sugar and liquorice.

Life Everlasting: Gnaphalium Polycephalium
PART USED: The herb
Hot fomentations of the herb have been used like arnica for sprains and bruises. Dried flowers have been used for a pillow for TB patients. Ulcerations of the mouth and throat are

relieved by chewing the leaves and blossoms. A warm infusion is very good for fevers, for quinsy and also bronchial and pulmonary complaints. Life everlasting and liquorice root chewed are said to be good for singers and speakers.

Lily of the Valley: Convallaria majalis
PART USED: Root
Mucilaginous

Strengthens the brain, makes thoughts clearer. Extremely useful in dropsy, epilepsy, dizziness, convulsions, palsy and apoplexy. Is quieting to the heart.

Lobelia: Lobelia inflata
PART USED: Plant and seed
Emetic, expectorant, diuretic, nervine, diaphoretic, anti-spasmodic

A powerful relaxant. Lobelia alone cannot cure, but is beneficial with other herbs. Pleurisy root is good for pleurisy, but is better still if combined with lobelia. Catnip added to lobelia for an enema. Add lobelia to poultices. Lobelia is excellent for nervous patients and as an emetic. Also excellent in whooping-cough remedies. For hepatitis, use equal parts of pleurisy root, catnip and bitter root. Lobelia reduces excitability of heart (angina pectoris). A good combination is lobelia seed, lady slipper and capsicum (cayenne). Is a good remedy for laryngitis. Also for scarlet fever, chickenpox, measles, smallpox and diphtheria. Excellent for lock-jaw. One tablespoonful of the tincture is used for asthma, taken every ten minutes for three doses if necessary. A tincture is made with half ounce lobelia herb, two ounces of the seed (crushed), one tablespoonful cayenne and one quart cider vinegar. Macerate ten days to two weeks in a stoppered bottle. Shake every day. An antispasmodic tincture for pain or lock-jaw is made as follows: Crushed lobelia seed, skullcap, skunk cabbage, gum myrrh, black cohosh, one ounce each and one-half ounce cayenne. Infuse in one pint of alcohol for one week, shaking well daily. Keep closely stoppered. Dose—one teaspoonful in one-half cup warm water.

Mandrake: Podophyllum peltatum (May Apple)
PART USED: Root
Antibilious, cathartic, emetic, diaphoretic, cholagogue, alterrative, resolvent, vermifuge, deobstruent.

Excellent liver and bowel regulator. Combine with senna. Has no equal in chronic liver disorders. Very beneficial to uterine diseases. Acts upon all tissues and cells of the body. Valuable in hepatitis. One teaspon to one pint of boiling water—one teaspoon of the tea at a time. Good in typhoid fever. A fine remedy when properly given in small doses.

Marigold: Calendula
PART USED: Flowers and leaves
Useful externally and internally for cancers, wounds, ulcers, hepatitis and amenorrhoea. Makes an excellent salve. Tincture made of the marigold flowers acts like tincture of arnica for bruises and sprains. It is little less effectual in smallpox and measles than saffron.

Marjoram: Origanum marhorana
PART USED: Whole plant.
Aromatic, tonic, condiment, emmenagogue

A good tonic. A good combination with camomile and gentian. Poultice very beneficial for sprains, felons, boils, carbuncles. Good for loss of appetite, eruptive diseases, suppressed menstruation. Expels gas. Increases flow of urine. Is good in hepatitis, deafness, headache, indigestion, nausea, colic, neuralgia. Oil dropped in cavity of aching tooth is said to stop pain. Will expel poisons from the body.

Milkweed: Asclepias syriaca
PART USED: Root
Emetic, purgative, alterative, diuretic, tonic
Splendid for female trouble, bowel and kidney trouble. Increases flow of urine. Good in dropsy, asthma, stomach trouble. Combined with marshmallow (equal parts), four cups daily. Will remove gallstones in a short time.

Mistletoe: Viscum flavescens—viscum album
PART USED: Young twigs and leaves
Narcotic, antispasmodic, emetic, tonic, nervine

I

Excellent for cholera, St. Vitus Dance, epilepsy, convulsions. hysteria, delirium, nervous debility and heart trouble.

Motherwort: Leonurus cardiaca
PART USED: Tops and leaves
Antispasmodic, nervine, emmenagogue, laxative, hepatic
Excellent results in female trouble. Useful in cramp, convulsions, hysteria, sleeplessness, delirium tremens, liver disorders, suppressed urine, colds (especially chest colds). Increases menstrual flow. Has excellent effect if taken during pregnancy. Expels worms. Strengthens the heart—two tablespoonfuls of the infusion every two hours. An excellent aid to digestion when taken at mealtime. A hot fomentation wrung out of strong tea will relieve cramp of menstruation.

Mullein: Verbascum thapsus
PART USED: Leaves and root
Anodyne, diuretic, demulcent, antispasmodic, vulnerary, stringent, emollient, pectoral
For asthma, burn root and inhale fumes. A tea of the leaves is useful in asthma, croup, bronchitis, all lung ailments, bleeding from lungs, difficult breathing, hay fever. Makes a good gargle. Will induce sleep and relieve pain. Fomentation wrung out of hot tea is good applied to mumps, tumours, sore throat, tonsilitis. Crushed fresh flowers said to remove warts. The tea is excellent for dropsy, sinusitis, swollen joints. One ounce boiled in a pint of water or soy milk, one-half teacupful after each bowel movement for diarrhoea. Fomentations good for prostate swellings, swellings of any kind, bad sores. A syrup made with mullein leaves good for irritating coughs. Also good for sciatica, spinal soreness, inflammatory rheumatism. Tincture of mullein combined with tincture of black cohosh and lobelia used in liniments. Poultice of mullein, lobelia and black cohosh will give relief in neuralgia. Ointment of mullein for haemorrhoids as well as the tea taken internally. Fresh leaves in vinegar also a good application to mumps and other swellings. For bad colds, drink hot on retiring.

Myrrh: Balsamodendron myrrh
PART USED: Powdered gum

Antiseptic, stimulant, tonic, expectorant, vulnerary, em-menagogue

A valuable tonic. Good in bronchial and lung diseases. Is said to remove halitosis (bad breath) when taken internally. For sick stomach, a small teaspoon of the powdered gum and of golden seal to a pint of boiling water, one teaspoon of the infusion six times a day. Made into an ointment with golden seal is excellent injected into rectum for haemorrhoids. Good for gangrene and as a mouth-wash. An excellent gargle for diphtheria, sore throat and sores in the mouth. Infusion is also good for coughs, asthma, and all chest complaints. Diminishes mucous discharges. A few drops of infusion give instant temporary relief in toothache. Two ounces of tincture of myrrh and one-half ounce of cayenne to a quart of alcohol makes the best antiseptic. Taken (a few drops in a glass of water), is a powerful stimulant in shock, collapse and prostration.

Nettle: Urtica Dioca, Stinging Nettle
PART USED: Root and leaves
Pectoral, duretic, astringent, tonic, styptic, rubifacient

Nettles contain iron, sulphur, potassium and sodium. Nettles are excellent for kidney trouble. They expel bladder stones, increase flow of urine. Also excellent in a reducing diet when used with seawrack. The boiled leaves applied externally will stop bleeding almost at once. A poultice of the green leaves will relieve pain, but will blister if left on too long. Good in diarrhoea, will expel worms. Tea of the root is used in dropsy, in the first stages, in haemorrhaging from urinary organs, lungs, intestines, stomach and nose. Tea from leaves will clean out urinary tract. Will also expel phlegm from lungs. Excellent hair tonic. Will bring back natural colour. Also removes dandruff. Simmer for thirty minutes. Use as a final rinse after shampoo. Massage well into scalp. Leaves may be boiled in vinegar for the same results. The green leaves, cooked like spinach, make a good blood purifier. The prickles of the plant contain formic acid. Seeds and flowers macerated in wine are given for ague. Nettle will also increase the menstrual flow. A

strong cup of nettle, combined with wild cherry bark and
blackberry root, is especially helpful in summer complaint
of children and bowel trouble of adults. A man of 80 years in
England attributed his third set of molars to having eaten
nettles and dandelion leaves. These may have helped, but other
food factors than are found in these two herbs would be necessary to grow a third set of teeth. General nutrition as well as
the forming of teeth is dependent upon the maintenance of a
proper ratio betwen calcium and phosphorus. Neither nettles
nor dandelion leaves contain phosphorus.

Orris: Germanica, pallida, Florentine Iris
PART USED: Root
Fresh leaves have little or no scent. Characteristic violet
odour is gradually developed during drying process. Maximum
fragrance is reached after two years.

Papaya: a tropical fruit, has no equal for stomach and bowe
ailments.

Parsley: Petroselinum sativum
PART USED: Root, leaves and seed
Diuretic, aperient, expectorant. Juice is antiperiodic. Seed is
febrifuge and emmenagogue.
Roots and leaves are excellent for difficult urination,
hepatitis, fevers, obstruction of liver and spleen. For female
trouble, combine leaves with equal parts of buchu, crampbark
and black haw. Hot fomentation is applied to insect bites and
stings. Poultice of bruised leaves is excellent for swollen glands,
swollen breasts. Will dry up milk. A tea from the crushed seeds
will kill head lice. Excellent for dropsy, which may follow
scarlatina or other similar diseases. Parsley is excellent to
inhibit cancer. Parsley is rich in potassium. It has been found
that cancer cells cannot multiply in potassium.

Peach: Amygdalus persica
PART USED: Bark, leaves, twigs and kernels
Relaxant, demulcent, sedative, laxative, aromatic
Exert excellent influence over nervous system. Good results
in whooping cough and hepatitis. Expels worms. Effective for

nausea in preganancy. Excellent for bladder and uterine ailments. Taken hot in small doses (large swallow every hour or two) will stop vomiting in cholera morbus. Powdered bark or leaves heals sores. Kernels, bruised and boiled in vinegar (cider) until they become thick are said to be excellent for baldness and to grow hair. Peach leaves are more effective than quinine for purposes for which quinine is used, and is harmless. Tea from leaves is a soothing tonic to the stomach. DO NOT LET STAND OVERNIGHT, since prussic acid forms on fermentation. Combine peach leaves with juniper berries or other strong diuretics.

Pennyroyal: Hedeoma Pulegioides
PART USED: Whole plant
Sudorific, carminative, emmenagogue, stimulant, diaphoretic, aromatic, sedative

Excellent in fevers. Will promote perspiration, taken hot. Effective in gout, phlegm in chest and lungs, leprosy, hepatitis, dropsy, headache, colic, griping cramps, scanty menstruation brought on by colds. Bathe feet in hot water. Will relieve nausea but should not be taken during pregnancy. Good as a poultice or a wash for bruises and black eyes. Good for nervousness, skin diseases. The oil of pennroyal, combined with other essential oils, is used in liniment. A few drops of oil of pennyroyal rubbed on face and hands is a safeguard against mosquitoes. The oil mixed with raw linseed oil is effective for burns. The tea relieves spasms, hysterics, promotes expectoration in TB and coughs, whooping cough. Upon taking a cold, drink freely of the hot tea. Will ward off bad effects, fever, etc. In drying this herb, tie in bunches and hang in warm dry, shady place. It loses its strength fast when exposed to the air.

Peppermint: Mentha piperita
PART USED: Whole plant
Aromatic, stimulant, stomachic, carminative. Oil is stimulant and rubefacient.

Excellent for chills, fevers, gas on stomach, nausea, vomiting diarrhoea, cholera, heart trouble, 'flu and colds, and hysteria.

Applied externally (the oil) for rheumatism, neuralgia and headache. Peppermint enemas are excellent in cholera and colon trouble, convulsions and spasms in infants. Helpful in cases of insanity. Hot, strong peppermint tea will restore one after fainting or dizzy spells. Good for griping from eating unripe fruit or irritating foods. Strengthens heart muscles. Cleanses and strengthens the entire body. Use a hot peppermint tea in place of aspirin for headache. Take a cupful of the hot tea, lie down for a while and relax and your headache will be gone. Strengthens the nerves. Taken with meals, will assist digestion. Use a few drops of the essence in water if leaves are not on hand. The oil is also used for toothache. Also used in flavouring. A protection against seasickness.

Plantain: Plantago major
PART USED: Whole plant.
Alterative, diuretic, antisyphilitic, antiseptic, astringent, de-obstruent, styptic, vulnerary.

The American Indians used this herb. Both the narrow and wide leaf are good. Has a soothing, cooling, healing effect on sores, ulcers and burns. Fresh leaves (crushed) will check bleeding. Useful for erysipelas, eczema, burns and scalds. Make a strong tea and apply often. Inject the tea for haemorrhoids after each stool. For haemorrhoids, boil the herb slowly about two hours in soy bean oil or other good vegetable oil. For leucorrhoea, use a strong tea as a douche. Especially valuable for diarrhoea, kidney and bladder trouble, pain in lumbar area, bed wetting. The green leaves (bruised) are applied as a poultice for stings by poisonous insects, snake bites, tumours, carbuncles and boils. Will ease pain in bowels. Will clear head of mucous. Used effectively for dropsy. A tea made with distilled water is used for a wash for inflamed eyes. Expels worms. Equal parts of plantain and yellow dock make an excellent wash for running sores, ringworm, and impetigo. Also excellent in salve for new or old sores.

Pleurisy: Asclepias Tuberosa
PART USED: Root

Expectorant, carminative, tonic, diuretic, diaphoretic, relaxant, antispasmodic

Valuable in pleurisy. Excellent for colds, flu, bronchial and pulmonary ailments. Very useful in scarlet fever, rheumatism, fevers, lung fever, typhus and measles. Clean stomach first with an emetic. Apply a cold compress to area and cover with a flannel for pleurisy. Pleurisy root is a good kidney tonic and is effective in asthma. For peritonitis, combine with a very small amount of lobelia. Promotes perspiration and expectoration in diseases of the respiratory tract. Also found valuable in uterine ailments.

Poke Root: Phytolacca decandra
PART USED: Root
Alterative, resolvent, deobstruent, detergent, antisyphilitic, antiscorbutic

Tender leaves in early spring make excellent greens. Tones up the whole system. The root makes a good spring tonic. The root excites the whole glandular system. Best alterative known. The green root is especially good for enlargement of the glands and spleen, especially the thyroid gland. For goitre, take internally and apply externally. Tea is excellent in eczema and other skin diseases and impetigo. Good as a poultice for caked breast.

Prickly Ash: Xanthoxylum
PART USED: Bark and berries
Stimulant, tonic, alterative, sialagogue

As a stimulant in languid states of the system. Has proved effective in paralysis of the tongue and mouth, for rheumatism, hepatitis. Berries are stimulant, carminative, anti-spasmodic, acting especially on the mucous membranes. Will increase flow of saliva. If taken on an irritable stomach, may cause vomiting. For numbness and poor circulation.

Psylla: Plantago psyllium
PART USED: Seed
Demulcent, purgative, detergent

Excellent in cases of colitis, ulcers and haemorrhoids.

Cleanses the intestines of toxins, taken one hour before meals (one or two teaspoonfuls in half glass of hot water). For children, half to one teaspoonful. Vary dose according to need. Lubricates as well as it cleans out colon.

Red Clover: Trifolium pratense
PART USED: Blossoms
Depurative, detergent, alterative, mild stimulant

Wonderful blood purifier. Combined with equal parts of violet leaves and flowers, burdock, yellow dock, dandelion root, rock rose and golden seal, it has proved a powerful agent in growths, leprosy and pellagra. Used alone it has proven valuable in bronchial coughs and whooping cough. Warm tea is soothing to the nerves. Healing to fresh wounds and burns. Excellent in salve. A good formula is made by combining one ounce red clover blossoms, one ounce burdock seed, two ounces Oregon grape root and half ounce blood root. Steep in one pint hot water and one pint hot apple cider for two hours. A small glassful four times a day. Has proven good in cases of growths in any part of the body. If in the throat, gargle four or five times a day. If in the stomach, drink frequently through the day. If in the rectum, inject with a syringe. If in the uterus, use as a douche, holding vagina closed and lie with upper part of body lower. Hold as long as possible. I have seen growths and tumours disappear when an ointment was made thus: Make a very strong tea of red clover blossoms, and violet leaves and flowers. Strain, simmer tea slowly until it looks like black tar and is of the consistency of tar. Violet leaves and flowers added to red clover blossoms make them an even greater specific for growths. In his book, *Medicinal Value of Natural Foods*. Dr. W. H. Graves lists red clover as being helpful in jaundice, skin diseases, anaemia, constipation, nervous exhaustion, and aids the eradication of destructive drug poisons from the body. It is also suited to the respiratory organs, thus is beneficial in whooping cough, asthma and other respiratory ailments.

Red Raspberry: Rubus stringosus
PART USED: Leaves

Anti-emetic, astringent, purgative, stomachic, parturient, tonic, stimulant and alterative

Fruit is laxative, anti-acid, parturient, esculent.

Will remove cankers from mucous membranes. Excellent for diarrhoea, especially in infants. Decreases menstrual flow without stopping it abruptly. Will allay nausea. Very good astringent. An aid to labour if combined with spikenard and taken the last six weeks of pregnancy.

Red Root: Ccanothus Americanus

PART USED: Bark of the root

Astringent, expectorant, sedative

Excellent for spleen trouble. Gargle every two hours with a strong tea of red root for badly enlarged tonsils. Inject strong tea for haemorrhoids.

Rhubarb: Rheum palmatium

PART USED: Root

Vulnerary, tonic, stomachic, purgative, astringent, aperient

Excellent laxative for infants. A mild tonic. Excellent to increase muscular action of the bowels. Good in stomach trouble. Relieves headache. Effective in liver disorders. The powdered root is a valuable and prompt cathartic. A splendid diuretic for children.

Rock Rose: Helianthemum Canadense

PART USED: Herb and oil

Aromatic, tonic, alterative, astringent

Oil most valuable part. Superior physic for cancer. Excellent gargle for cankered sore throat and scarlatina. Good for diarrhoea. A valuable remedy in combination with corydalis, formosa and stillingia.

Rosemary: Rosemarinus officinalis

PART USED: Leaves and flowers

Stimulant, antispasmodic, emmenagogue, tonic, astringent, diaphoretic, carminative, nervine, aromatic, cephalic

Old-fashioned remedy for colds, colic, nervous ailments. Very good for nervous headache. Good mouth-wash for gums, halitosis, sore throat. Helpful in insanity. Aids digestion, cough.

Strengthens the eyes. Oil used for ointments, liniment and in perfumery. Helps a weak memory, quickens the senses, clears the vision. Best hair rinse. Drink hot morning and night for rheumatism and arthritis. Must persevere in its use.

Rue: Ruta Graveolens
PART USED: Whole plant
Aromatic, pungent, tonic, emmenagogue, stimulant, antispasmodic

Relieves congestion of the uterus. Stimulant and tonic effect. For painful menstruation. Excellent remedy for the stomach, cramp, nervousness, hysteria, convulsions, dizziness, insanity. Expels worms. Relieves headache. Excellent for colic convulsions in children. Poultice good for sciatica, joint pain and gout. It resists poisons. The seed in wine (tincture) an antidote against all dangerous medicines and deadly poisons. Good for the elderly. Preserves ordinary vision.

Saffron: Carthamus tinctorius
PART USED: Flowers and seed
Laxative, emmenagogue, condiment, carminative, sudorific, diuretic, diaphoretic. Seed is aromatic, laxative and diuretic

One of the most reliable remedies in measles, scarlet fever, all skin diseases and other eruptive maladies. Produces profuse perspiration when taken hot. Useful in colds and 'flu. Regulates the menstrual flow.

Sage: Saliva officinalis
PART USED: Leaves
Sudorific, astringent, expectorant, tonic, aromatic, antispasmodic, nervine, vermifuge

Wounds heal more rapidly when washed with sage tea. Soothing to the nerves. Good for palsy. For quinsy and sore throat drink the tea and also gargle. Especially good mixed with lemon and honey. Expels worms. Will stop bleeding. Good in kidney and liver trouble. Effective in fevers, 'flu (taken hot). Will relieve pain in head. Will dry up breasts. Will make hair grow when hair roots are not destroyed. Removes dandruff. Good in joint pains. Excellent to strengthen the memory. Quickens the senses. Good when weaning a child.

For that reason it is not good if a woman hopes to breast feed her baby. Gives a quality of acute mental discernment.

Sanicle: Sanicula marilandica
PART USED: Root and leaves
Vulnerary, astringent, alterative, expectorant, discutient, depurative
Powerful to cleanse the body of mucous and poisonous waste matter.

Sarsaparilla: Smilax officinalis
PART USED: Root
Alterative, diuretic, demulcent, antispasmodic, stimulant, antiscorbutic
Excellent antidote for deadly poisons. Increases flow of urine. A good eyewash. Promotes profuse perspiration when taken hot. Good for infants infected with venereal disease. Sarsaparilla was the wonder drug of the gay '90s. In recent years renewed interest is being centred in this herb. Research has discovered that it contains organic hormones.

Sassafras: Laurus—Sassafras officinalis
PART USED: Inner bark of root
Aromatic, stimulant, alterative, diaphoretic and diuretic
Purifies blood, cleanses whole system. Will relieve gas. Valuable in colic and all skin diseases. Good wash for eyes. Good in kidney and bladder trouble. Good in varicose ulcers as a wash. Also take tea internally. A good tonic after childbirth. A rustic spring tonic. The oil of sassafras is excellent for toothache when applied to the aching tooth.

Skullcap: Scutellaria Lateriflora
PART USED: Whole plant
Nervine, tonic, antispasmodic
One of the best tonic nervines. Combined with cayenne and golden seal it cannot be surpassed for heart weakness. With lady slipper it is the best nerve tonic. Useful in hydrophobia and poisonous snake bites. Effective in delirium tremens, St. Vitus Dance, shaking palsy, convulsions. Equal parts of skullcap, nerve root, hops, catnip and black cohosh aids in

morphine addiction. Produces calm sleep. Also effective in lock-jaw, ague, fevers and neuralgia.

Sea Wrack: Fucus Vesiculosus, Bladder Wrack
PART USED: The dried plant
   Sea wrack is a seaweed. It is considered alterative. It is rich in organic minerals, being used chiefly as a blood purifier. It is the most important ingredient in the majority of obesity treatments and is harmless.

Shepherd's Purse: Capsella Bursa Pastoris
PART USED: Whole plant
   Stops bleeding in fifteen minutes. Contains vitamin K. Excellent in haemorrhages of all kinds.

Slippery Elm: Ulmus Fulva
PART USED: Inner bark
Demulcent, emollient, nutritive
   Useful in dysentery, diarrhoea, diseases of the urinary tract and bronchitis. The bark chewed will relieve heartburn. Externally, as a poultice, it is useful for inflammations, boils, etc. Also effective for rectal and vaginal suppositories. Chew and swallow the juice for minor sore throat. It is an antidote for many poisons. Acts the same as white of egg. Use the tea as an enema.

Sorrel: Rumex acetosa
PART USED: Leaves and root
Diuretic, antiscorbutic, refrigerant, vermifuge
   Leaves may be used as greens. Expels worms. Expels kidney stones. Good in hepatitis. Poultice is used for boils and tumours. Not active after drying. Contains acid potassium, oxalate and tartaric acid.

Southernwood: Artemisia abrotanum
PART USED: Leaves and tops
Leaves and tops have a strong fragrance. Said to be obnoxious to various insects. Drives away moths.

Spearmint: Mentha viridis
PART USED: Whole plant
Antispasmodic, aromatic, diuretic, diaphoretic, carminative

Good for colic, gas in stomach and bowels, spasms, dropsy, nausea and vomiting, bladder stones, relieves suppressed urine. Excellent as an application and injection for haemorrhoids. Effective for inflammation of kidneys and bladder. Excellent to stop vomiting in pregnancy. Soothing to the nerves. Never boil spearmint. Essence is added to nervine liniments.

Spikenard: Aralia racemosa
PART USED: Root
Pectoral, diaphoretic, stimulant, alterative, balsamic, expectorant
Eases childbirth if taken last six weeks of pregnancy. Excellent blood purifier. Good in all skin eruptions, pimples, etc. Useful in coughs, colds and chest troubles. Combined with red raspberry leaves for easy childbirth. Too much will cause headache. Good for joint pain. Breaks tough phlegm. Effective against bites of poisonous creatures.

Squaw Vine: Mitchella Repens
PART USED: Whole plant
Diuretic, astringent, tonic, alterative, parturient
Wonderful for easy, painless childbirth. Excellent for sore eyes, uterine troubles, female complaints. To bathe sore nipples, add a little olive oil or cream. Mother's Antispasmodic Compound #410, sold by Indiana Botanic Gardens, is especially good last six weeks of pregnancy. It contains squaw vine.

Strawberry: Fragaria vesca
PART USED: Leaves
Astringent, tonic, diuretic. Fruit is diuretic, refrigerant
Good for a beverage. Tones up the appetite and system. Good for bowel troubles. Cleanses the stomach. Excellent for children. Good for eczema, externally and internally. Good used in an enema. Water made with the berries is used as a wash for eyes. Takes away film or skin that sometimes grows over the eyes.

Sumach: Rhus glabrum
PART USED: Berries, bark and leaves
Bark and leaves: tonic, astringent, alterative, antiseptic.

Berries: diuretic, refrigerant, emmenagogue, diaphoretic, cephalic

Used in combination of equal parts of sumach berries and bark, white pine bark and slippery elm bark. This tea is very cleansing to the system. Tea of the berries is excellent for bowel complaints, fevers, sores and cankers of mouth. Gargle and wash for sore mouth and sore throat. Bark of sumach makes an excellent wash for old sores. Tea of the berries is slightly acid and is good in cases of malarial fever.

Sweet Balm: Melissa officinalis
PART USED: Whole herb and flowers
Aromatic, emmenagogue, diaphoretic, cephalic

Excellent taken hot for fevers, colds and flu. Good for nausea and vomiting. Will quiet and settle the stomach. Good in kidney and bladder troubles, headache, suppressed urine, painful menstruation and female disorders. Lemon juice added to the hot tea is good in fevers and will promote perspiration.

Sweet Flag: Calamus
PART USED: Root
Stimulant, tonic

Improves gastric juices. Removes gas and sour stomach. Good in dropsy. Will prevent return of intermittent fever in marshy regions. A good stomach tonic. Increases the appetite. Stimulates digestion. Has an antiseptic effect upon gums and teeth. The Indians chewed the root for toothache. Chewing the root is said to clear the voice for singers and speakers.

Tansy: Tanacetum vulgare
PART USED: Whole herb.
Aromatic, tonic, emmenagogue, diaphoretic, vulnerary. Seed is vermifuge.

Good for dyspepsia. One of the best remedies to promote menstruation. Seeds will expel worms. Taken hot is excellent in fevers, ague, colds and 'flu. Strengthens weak veins (varicose veins). Hot fomentations are applied to swellings, tumours, inflammations, bruises, sciatica and inflamed eyes. Good remedy in heart disease. In small doses it is excellent in convalescence, hysteria and hepatitis. Oil of tansy rubbed on body repels insects.

Twin Leaf: Jeffersonia diphylla
PART USED: Root
Diuretic, alterative, antisyphilitic, antispasmodic, tonic
    Good gargle for sore throat. Fine for scarlatina, scarlet fever. Applied as a hot fomentation, it will relieve pain anywhere in the body. In severe pain take hot internally.

Unicorn: Aletris farimosa—Star Root
PART USED: Root
    Valuable tonic in general debility, hysteria and colic. Strengthens female organs. Protects against miscarriage. Good in chlorosis, engorged condition of the uterus. For prolapsus of the uterus (falling of the organ).

Uva Ursi: Arctostaphylos uva ursi
PART USED: Leaves
Diuretic
    Good in all kidney troubles. Excellent for excessive menstruation, for spleen, liver, pancreas ailments, mucous discharge from bladder with pus and blood. Excellent for ulceration of neck of womb and all female troubles. Use also as a douche.

Valerian: Valerian officinalis
PART USED: Root
Aromatic, stimulant, tonic, anodyne, antispasmodic, nervine
    Excellent nerve tonic. Valuable in hysteria. Taken hot will promote menstruation. Excellent for measles, scarlet fever, restlessness, convulsions in infants. Useful in colic, fevers. Will break up colds. Good for gravel in bladder. Heals ulcerated stomach. Powerful preventive of fermentation and gas. Do not boil root. A little peppermint increases promptness of action. Excites the cerebro-spinal system. In large doses it will cause headache. Valerian added to boiled liquorice, raisins and anise seed is good for cough, shortness of breath and to expectorate phlegm. Eases pain. Promotes sleep.

Vervain: Verbena hastata
PART USED: Whole plant
Tonic, sudorific, expectorant, vulnerary, emetic, nervine, emmenagogue, vermifuge

Powerful to promote profuse perspiration. Excellent in fevers. Will often cure colds overnight. Excellent in whooping cough, pneumonia, asthma, ague. Expels phlegm from throat and chest. Good in all female troubles. Will increase the menstrual flow. Expels worms. Useful in nervousness, delirium, insanity, sleeplessness, nervous headache. Will tone up system convalescing from heart disease. Shortness of breath, wheezing, asthma. Excellent in cases of appendicitis. Healing to sores. One part vervain, two parts wahoo and two parts butternut bark, made into a syrup, is valuable for chronic constipation in malarial difficulties.

Violet: Clematis virginica
PART USED: Leaves and flowers
Stimulant, diuretic, sudorific, vesicant

Relieves severe headache. Combined with red clover blossoms and rock rose, and made into a poultice, is helpful in ulcers, bed sores and eruptive diseases.

Wahoo: Euonymus atropurpureus
PART USED: Bark of root
Tonic, laxative, expectorant, diuretic, alterative

A good laxative. Valuable in chest and lung ailments. Useful in torpid liver, fevers. Excellent influence on pancreas and spleen. Good for dropsy. Improves digestion. Is valuable when combined with gentian, golden seal. Breaks chills. Useful in constipation. Also in pulmonary ailments.

Water Pepper: Polygonum punctatum—Smart Weed
PART USED: Whole plant
Astringent, diaphoretic, tonic, stimulant, emmenagogue, antiseptic

For scanty menstruation. All uterine troubles, gravel in bladder, colds, coughs, bowel complaints, kidney disorders. Valuable in appendicitis. Use as enema and place hot fomentation to abdomen. Used as a wash in erysipelas. Use in cold water.

Wild Cherry: Prunus Virginiana.

PART USED: Inner bark

Mild tonic, sedative, pectoral, aromatic, astringent

Excellent in TB, bronchitis, fever, coughs which are loose. Do not use for dry coughs. Good for diarrhoea in children. Good in indigestion, asthma, colds and 'flu. Also good to reduce blood pressure. Do not boil wild cherry.

Wild Plum:

PART USED: Bark

Best remedy for asthma.

White Willow: Salix alba

PART USED: Bark, leaves and buds

Febrifuge, antiperiodic

Good in heartburn, all kinds of fevers, chills, ague, acute rheumatism. Tea made from leaves or buds is used in gangrene, cancer, eczema. Good for bleeding wounds, nose bleed, spitting of blood. Also good as an eyewash. Increases flow of urine.

Wintergreen: Gaultheria Procumbens

PART USED: Leaves

Stimulant, antiseptic, astringent, diuretic, emmenagogue, cardiac depressant

Taken in small frequent doses will stimulate stomach, heart and respiratory tract. Good in rheumatic fever, sciatica, all bladder troubles and skin diseases. Valuable in colic. Expels gas. Good for dropsy, cystitis, stomach troubles, bowel obstructions. Oil is valuable in liniments. Poultice is good for boils, swellings, ulcers and felons. Good as a douche for leucorrhoea. Also for gargle for sore throat. Good wash for sore eyes. Large doses may cause vomiting. Indians used wintergreen berries as a very invigorating drink for the stomach. Wintergreen has a far-reaching effect. Penetrates every cell. Acts on cause of pain. For arthritis and rheumatism, the following recipe has proved effective. Using the oil of wintergreen, begin with one drop, three times a day, the first day. Two drops three times a day the second day. Increase the drops one each day

K

until nine drops are taken. Then decrease a drop each day
until none are taken.

Witch Hazel: Hamamelis Virginica
PART USED: Bark and leaves
Astringent, tonic, antiphlogistic, sedative
   Unsurpassed to stop excessive menstruation, haemorrhages
from lungs, stomach, uterus, bowels. Good in diarrhoea and
as an enema. For nose bleed, snuff tea up nose. Inject tea for
haemorrhoids. Will restore circulation. Excellent as a gargle.

Wood Betony: Betonica officinalis
PART USED: Leaves
Aperient, stomachic, nervine, tonic, antiscorbutic
   Excellent for headache, insanity, neuralgia, stomach trouble,
heartburn, indigestion, stomach cramp, hepatitis, palsy,
convulsions, gout, colic, nervous ailments, dropsy, colds, 'flu,
poisonous bites. Expels worms. Opens obstructions of spleen
and liver. A good formula is two parts wood betony, one part
skullcap, one part sweet flag. It is a valuable herb.

Wood sage: Teucrium scorodonia
PART USED: Whole plant
Tonic, vermifuge, alterative, diuretic, slightly diaphoretic.
Improves appetite. Good wash for sores combined with chickweed. Used as a poultice for tumours combined with comfrey
and ragwort. Useful in quinsy, sore throat, colds, fevers, palsy,
kidney and bladder ailments. Increases flow of urine and also
the menstrual flow.

Yarrow: Achillea millefolium—Milfoil
PART USED: Whole plant
Astringent, tonic, alterative, diuretic, vulnerary
   Excellent for bleeding from the lungs. If the tea is taken
freely at the beginning of a cold, mixed with elderberry blossoms
and peppermint, and one remains in bed, it will break up a cold
in twenty-four hours. Yarrow is also useful in eruptive diseases
such as measles, chickenpox and smallpox. It has a very healing
and soothing effect on the mucous membranes. Yarrow is

especially useful in making a healing salve or ointment for all wounds. Is good in typhoid. Excellent in diarrhoea in infants and for uterine ailments. Expels gas. Is excellent as a douche for leucorrhoea. It is said to be good for falling hair if the head is bathed in the decoction. It contains a trace of sulphur.

Yellow Dock: Rumex crispus
PART USED: Root
Alterative, tonic, depurative, astringent, antiscorbutic, detergent

Tones up entire system. Good in eruptive diseases, swellings, leprosy, and as an eyewash. Also for impetigo (as an ointment). Excellent blood purifier. Helpful in glandular disorders.

Yerba Santa: Eriodyction glutinosum
PART USED: Leaves
Tonic, expectorant

Good in chronic laryngitis, bronchitis, asthma. Useful when there is excessive discharge from the nose. Good for rheumatism. Used as a tonic.

Yerba Reuma—as an application for shingles.

Yerba Mate

Some suggest using yerba mate in a reducing diet. It is supposed to lessen the feeling of hunger without fattening elements. Gives strength and endurance. Produces mental exhilaration with no subsequent organic or physical destruction. It is more stimulating than tea or coffee. Contains more chlorophyll than green or black tea. Under stress and strain, may be temporarily used as a substitute for solid food. Mate leaves contain 0.2 to 2% theine, a stimulating principle. Chinese tea contains from 1 to 5%. Mate contains far less tannin, an astringent principle, than Chinese tea.

CHAPTER XVIII

Medical Terms

ALTERATIVE A medicine which works a gradual healthy change and restoration of healthy functioning of all the organs.

ANODYNE Relieves pain.

ANTHELMINTIC Expels worms.

ANTHILITIC Prevents formation of calculi (stones) in the urinary organs..

ANTI-ACID Counteracts acidity of stomach and bowels.

ANTI-BILIOUS Relieves biliousness.

ANTI-EMETIC Stops vomiting.

ANTI-EPILEPTIC Relieves fits and epileptic seizures.

ANTI-PERIODIC Arrests morbid periodical movements.

ANTI-RHEUMATIC Relieves or cures rheumatism.

ANTI-SCORBUTIC Cures or prevents scurvy.

ANTISEPTIC Opposed to putrefaction.

ANTI-SPASMODIC Relieves or prevents spasms.

ANTI-SYPHILITIC Cures venereal diseases.

AROMATIC Spicy, flavours.

ASTRINGENT Causes contractions and arrests discharges.

CARMINATIVE Expels gas from bowels.

CATHARTIC Evacuates bowels.

CEPHALIC Used in diseases of the head.

CHOLAGOGUE Increases flow of bile.

CONDIMENT Improves flavour of food.

DEMULCENT Soothing, relieves inflammation.

DEOBSTRUENT Removes obstructions.

DEPURATIVE Purifies the blood.

DETERGENT Cleansing to boils, ulcers and wounds.

DIAPHORETIC Produces perspiration.

DISCUTIENT Dissolves and removes tumours.

DIURETIC Increases flow of urine.

EMETIC Produces vomiting.

EMMENAGOGUE Promotes menstruation.

EMOLLIENT Softens and soothing to inflamed parts.

EPISPASTIC Causes blisters.

ERRHINES Applied to membrane of nostrils, causes discharge.

ESCULENT Edible as food.

EXANTHEMATOUS Remedy for skin eruptions.

EXPECTORANT Capable of facilitating excretion of mucous from the chest.

FEBRIFUGE Reduces fever.

HEPATIC Remedy for diseases of the liver.

LAXATIVE Promotes bowel action.

LITHONTRYPTIC Dissolves calculi (stones) in the urinary organs.

MATURATING Ripens or brings boils, etc., to a head.

MUCILAGINOUS Soothing to inflamed parts.

NARCOTIC Diminishes action of nervous and vascular system, inducing sleep.

NAUSEANT Produces vomiting.

NERVINE Allays nervous excitement.

OPTHALMICUM Remedy for diseases of the eye.

PARTURIENT Induces and promotes labour at childbirth.

PECTORAL Remedy to relieve chest congestion.

REFRIGERANT Cooling.

RESOLVENT Dissolves and removes tumours.

RUBIFACIENT Increases circulation—produces red skin.

SEDATIVE Quieting to nerves.

SIALAGOGUE Increases secretion of saliva.

STOMACHIC Strengthens and gives tone to stomach.

STYPTIC Arrests haemorrhage and bleeding.

SUDORIFIC Produces perspiration.

TONIC Remedy which invigorates and strengthens.

VERMIFUGE Expels worms.

VULNERARY Healing to wounds.

CHAPTER XIX

When and How to Gather Herbs

THERE is a right time to gather medicinal plants.

Gather leaves in the morning after the dew is off, in clear, dry weather. To dry leaves, spread out thinly on a clean surface. Stir occasionally until thoroughly dry.

In collecting herbs, strip off the flowers, leaves and very small stems. The thick woody stems have no value. Dry same as leaves.

Collect flowers immediately upon opening, when they are of the best value. Dry with care to preserve their natural colour.

Barks may be gathered either in the spring or fall. The rough outer bark must be scraped off before peeling the inner bark. Barks may be dried in sunlight with the exception of wild cherry bark.

Seeds should be collected as soon as they are ripe. Only fully developed seeds have value. Remove any of no value.

CHAPTER XX

Cooking with Herbs

COOKING with herbs can be an adventure. It is also an art. It is fascinating to experiment with culinary herbs. Just a pinch of this or that will give you a dish fit for a king. And what woman doesn't cook for her king every day.

When you become skilled in using culinary herbs, you will be able to know secrets that will transform cheap cuts of meat, ordinary soup or salad into an epicurean delight.

Flavour is the secret of good cooking. The important thing is to use only a very small amount. If you were to use too much of any culinary herb, it would give you a foul-tasting, bitter dish that may destroy your desire to cook with herbs. Never let the herbal flavour dominate the dish.

There are many herbs that can be used culinary purposes.

THYME is a popular herb. It can be used in soups, especially in onion soup. It blends with chopped meats, roasts, steaks and chops. Also cheese dishes, carrots, peas, onions, steamed potatoes and fish stews can be enhanced by the use of thyme.

DILL may be used with cheese and egg dishes. Fish and sea foods, meat, salads, vegetable stews can all be made tasty with the addition of a small amount of dill.

FENNEL is used in breads, rolls, cakes and cookies, candies and confections. Can also be used in fish, meat and egg dishes, in soups and salads. It is delicious in sweet pickles.

ROSEMARY adds a delicious flavour to fricassees, roast beef and roast lamb. Can also be used in soups and sausage. Try it in fruit-salad dressing.

OREGANO is not too well known (pronounced o reg' an o). It is also called Mexican sage. It is very much like marjoram. Chili is improved by the addition of oregano. Try it in stews, gravies and sauces. It is used today in pizza cooking.

ALLSPICE resembles a mixture of cloves, cinnamon and nutmeg. Good in preserving, baking and pickling.

ANISE SEED is a flavour to tickle the palate of most people. It is used on cookies and coffee cake and in candies. It is a Christmas baking favourite.

SWEET BASIL is popular in soups, vegetables, boiled meats and in tomato dishes.

BAY LEAVES (laurel) gives a good flavour to soups, meats, fricassees, potatoes, fish and pickles.

CARAWAY is delicious in rye bread, cottage cheese, cabbage slaw and sauerkraut.

CARDAMON SEED is a well-known flavour in Danish pastry, coffee cake, bread and rolls.

CELERY SEED or celery flakes makes soups, stuffings, cole slaw, potato salad and meat loaf something to talk about.

CORIANDER SEED makes cookies, cakes and candies especially delicious. May also be used in salads.

CUMIN SEED is an old spice. Try beef with chopped onions mixed with cumin. It is an ingredient of chili powder.

GARLIC is good in meat cooking, especially hamburger. Also in spaghetti dishes. Use very sparingly. May be used as garlic powder, garlic juice or garlic salt.

GINGER is popularly used in gingerbread, pickles and stewed and dried fruit. Some like chicken rubbed inside and out with powdered ginger mixed with butter.

MACE can be used in spice cake or to flavour whipped cream for dessert topping.

MARJORAM may be used in stews, soups, sausage and with lamb and mutton.

ONION POWDER or flakes is too well known to elaborate on.

PAPRIKA is good used in salads and cottage cheese.

PARSLEY should be used as a food and not only as a garnish. It is a must in potato soup.

RED PEPPER (cayenne) in butter sauces used on cooked vegetables is good.

SAFFRON gives a rich golden tint and oriental flavour to rice dishes. Also to cakes, breads and rolls.

SAGE is well known, but its use should be encouraged. Used

in sausage, fish and in poultry stuffing. Pork roast is made especially tasty by the addition of sage.

SAVOURY in scrambled eggs is delicious.

SESAME and SUNFLOWER SEEDS are delicious used in candy, cookies, rolls, biscuits and breads.

TARRAGON has a distinctive flavour for beef, lamb and chicken. Make tarragon vinegar as follows. Wash herbs well. Place in a pint jar. Mix vinegar and salt and pour over herbs in jar. Cover tightly and store in refrigerator. Let stand overnight. Shake well in the morning and strain, and use in making salad dressings. Thyme, dill, fennel, mint, basil, sorrel, lemon balm and borage may also be used to make herb vinegar.

TUMERIC is used with ginger in pickling, especially in chow-chow and piccalilli. A little tumeric in creamed eggs and on sea foods is tasty.

Culinary herbs give cooking lip-smacking goodness. However, remember, for the best results USE SPARINGLY. Give only an extra touch to your cooking.

Serve dandelion greens raw with a lemon French dressing. Top with alternate layers of sliced orange and mild Bermuda onion slice.

Chopped chives add a good flavour to cottage cheese, potatoes, salads, sandwiches, soups, stews, meat and gravies.

The scum which rises on top of pickles can be remedied by putting a slice or two of horseradish root in the jar, which will sink to the bottom, taking all the scum with it.

Add a squeeze of lemon to your steaks. It brings out all the flavour.

Use sour cream instead of sweet milk when mashing potatoes and beat hard. Add chives for flavour.

Sumac–elderberry jelly. Boil one pint sumac berries in three pints of water until one quart of juice remains. Boil one quart of elderberries in three pints of water until soft. Strain both juices through cheese cloth. Mix and measure and add sugar, equal parts of juice and sugar. Proceed as for jelly making.

Sprinkle a little sage over a salad. It strengthens the memory.

Use young nettle sprouts and tops in the spring as a pot herb. Boiling renders the stinging hairs harmless.

Ground fennel sprinkled on food will prevent gas in the stomach and bowels from forming and will add a different, delicious taste.

The young shoots of angelica (masterwort) are steeped in honey or sugar, candied and crystallized or made up as a preserve the same as rhubarb.

Lemonade can be made with lemon balm (fresh).

Indians boiled the thick roots of pleurisy root for food. They prepared a crude sugar from the flowers and ate the young seed pods after boiling them with buffalo meat.

Agar-agar may be used like gelatine.

Marshmallow roots (fresh and dried) have a pleasant flavour similar to the confection sold under the name "Marshmallow".

Borage leaves taste similar to cucumbers and are tasty in salads.

Thyme is good as a beverage and helps to prevent colds and infection.

The tender leaves of lambsquarters. dandelion greens and the docks are used as salad greens as well as for pot herbs. The sour leaves of red-tip sorrel are delicious in salads. A persistent weed common in many gardens is purslane. It, too, is a good salad green.

There are many flowers that are good to eat either in salad or tea. Nasturtium blossoms are spicy and delicious. The leaf and blossoms of the pansy are a relishing addition to a salad. Shepherd's purse is also good as fresh young greens.

The berries of horse or bull nettle will curd milk in cheese making.

Jerusalem artichoke, which is really a wild sunflower, has a delicious tuber growing on its roots. It may be boiled, baked or roasted.

The roots of cat-tails my be eaten in the autumn, the tender shoots in the spring.

The roots and nut-like seeds of the American lotus may be eaten in the autumn. The roots may be eaten raw, baked or roasted.

Stinging nettle may be used as other greens in the spring or early summer.

Wild leeks may be used in the spring in any way in which onions are used. Try leek soup, it is delicious.

Gather the young shoots of the common broad-leafed milkweed. They may be cooked as you would asparagus. They are delicious buttered or creamed.

A tasty dessert may be made by boiling calamus root in honey or sugar syrup for several hours. It is a natural candy with an agreeable taste.

Horehound candy: Steep (not boil) two ounces of dried horehound in one and a half pints of water for thirty minutes. Strain and add honey and boil over a brisk fire until it hardens in cold water. Pour into a greased pan and cut into squares.

Dandelions and other so-called weeds may be a chief source of worry in your lawn or garden, but they are especially healthful. Long before your cultivated garden stuff is ready to use, these greens are especially plentiful.

However, there are many poisonous plants. Therefore, be absolutely certain of the identity of a plant before you use it for food.

If the full and proper use is made of the herb in the kitchen, it will not be required in the sickroom.

Make use of the culinary herbs. It is an art which can be both beneficial and profitable. It can help your health and your pocket-book.

CHAPTER XXI

Plant a Herb Garden

RESERVE a corner of your garden for a herb garden. Choose a spot with lots of sunshine.

You will be delighted with a mint bed. It can take over your garden though. Clip off the runners. You will find plenty of use for peppermint and spearmint. No beverage is complete without mint.

No garden should be without parsley. Use it freely and not just as a garnish. Parsley seeds take a long time to germinate, so be patient.

Other culinary herbs you will want to plant in your herb garden are thyme, chives, basil, dill, borage, sage, caraway, anise, marjoram, rosemary, winter and summer savoury, fennel, watercress, camomile, horehound, lavender, liquorice, pennyroyal, and rue.

You should try planting comfrey. It adds to any herb tea. Tarragon will also please you.

Try planting a few flowers for food. They will yield a fragrance unheard of. You might want to try pickled nasturtiums or a violet or rose conserve. Marigolds, violets and peonies may also be used as food. The ancient Egyptians used rosewater in their pies. Your apple and cherry pies will have a different flavour and you will like it. The Arabs made a sherbet of violets. Middle English folks pickled and preserved the gillyflowers. In the past, the rose was classed as a culinary vegetable.

If you do not have room for a garden, you can grow herbs in a window box the year round. A layer of gravel placed in the bottom of the box will help drainage.

Herbs are not difficult to grow. They need lots of sunshine. For the soil, use about one-third sand and a little fertilizer.

Herbs should not be overwatered. However, do not let your plants dry out either.

Culinary herbs are most flavourful just before they flower.

You may want to dry some of your herbs for winter use. Dried herbs should be sorted in tightly sealed glass jars. Dried herbs are three or four times stronger than fresh herbs.

Tansy can be planted in your herb garden. It drives off mosquitos, gnats and flies.

Watercress is a valuable food. A saying of the Greeks was "Eat watercress and learn more wit". Watercress served with a tart dressing and hard-boiled eggs is a meal in itself. Recent studies show that cress is rich in vitamins A and C. It also has a good supply of B-1 and B-2 and a small amount of E, also some iron and copper, calcium, phosphorus, sulphur and manganese. Watercress may also be grown in pots in the house for the winter months. The pot must have a hole at the bottom and the pot should fit into a larger pan of water which will supply plenty of water for the plant. Give plenty of sun and be sure the water container is always filled.

The month of May is a good time to plant a herb garden.

CHAPTER XXII

Miscellaneous

LIQUID MEASURE

2 teaspoonfuls = 1 tablespoonful

2 tablespoonfuls = 1 ounce

16 ounces = 1 pint

64 tablespoonfuls = 1 pint

128 teaspoonfuls = 1 pint

1 teaspoonful = about 1 fluid drachm (dram)

2 tablespoonfuls = about 1 fluid ounce

1 teacupful = about 4 fluid ounces

1 dram = 60 grains for weight or
60 minims (drops) for liquid measure

1 ounce = 8 drams

1 pound = 16 ounces for weight

1 pint = 16 ounces liquid measure

1 quart = 2 pints   ,,   ,,

1 gallon = 4 quarts   ,,   ,,

ABBREVIATIONS COMMONLY USED

Gamma = microgram (1/1000 of a milligram) mcg

mg = milligram

gm = gram

kg = kilogram (1000 grams)

gr = grain

U.S.P. Unit = U.S. Pharmacopoeia Unit

I.U. or Int. Unit = International Unit

In all cases of vitamin units the I.U. is the same as the U.S.P., with the exception of vitamin E, for which no U.S.P. unit has been established.

Two vitamins, B-1 and C, are commonly declared by weight and also by units. B-1 = 1 mg—U.S.P. or I.U. C = 1 mg—20 U.S.P. or I.U.

1000 micrograms (mcg) = 1 milligram (mg)
1000 milligrams = 1 gram
1000 grams = 1 kilogram
1 level teaspoonful = 5 cc (approximately)
1 level tablespoonful = 15 cc

To make an infusion, add the dried herb to boiling water. Cover and let steep until luke warm. A herb beverage is made in this way.

To make a decoction, instead of just steeping, let it boil slowly in a covered pan, usually from ten to twenty minutes.

For nose-bleed, lift arm on same side as nostril from which the blood flows above the head.

An old saying is that fennel seeds, leaves and root eaten is effective in obesity.

Elder flowers keep flies away.

Sassafras is an ant repellent.

Sweet white clover will keep moths out of clothing.

For peritonitis, try equal parts of marshmallow, slippery elm, sweet flag and dandelion root.

For fainting, place patient flat on back. Allow fresh air. Sprinkle face with cold water. Give lobelia, American valerian and cayenne.

For obesity take active exercise, keep bowels open, eat a fruit diet. Give the following combination of herbs—bladder wrack, mandrake, gentian root, spearmint.

Give pumpkin seed for bed-wetting.

For blood poisoning, grate red beet and apply as a poultice.

For a felon, place finger in a tea made of elecampane root as hot as can be borne. Or punch a hole in a lemon and place finger in it. A poultice of peach tree leaves is also said to be good.

For snoring, take six drops of olive oil and a pinch of dry mustard just before getting into bed.

MELVIN POWERS SELF-IMPROVEMENT LIBRARY

ASTROLOGY

____ASTROLOGY: HOW TO CHART YOUR HOROSCOPE *Max Heindel*   3.00
____ASTROLOGY: YOUR PERSONAL SUN-SIGN GUIDE *Beatrice Ryder*   3.00
____ASTROLOGY FOR EVERYDAY LIVING *Janet Harris*   2.00
____ASTROLOGY MADE EASY *Astarte*   3.00
____ASTROLOGY MADE PRACTICAL *Alexandra Kayhle*   3.00
____ASTROLOGY, ROMANCE, YOU AND THE STARS *Anthony Norvell*   4.00
____MY WORLD OF ASTROLOGY *Sydney Omarr*   5.00
____THOUGHT DIAL *Sydney Omarr*   4.00
____WHAT THE STARS REVEAL ABOUT THE MEN IN YOUR LIFE *Thelma White*   3.00

BRIDGE

____BRIDGE BIDDING MADE EASY *Edwin B. Kantar*   5.00
____BRIDGE CONVENTIONS *Edwin B. Kantar*   5.00
____BRIDGE HUMOR *Edwin B. Kantar*   3.00
____COMPETITIVE BIDDING IN MODERN BRIDGE *Edgar Kaplan*   4.00
____DEFENSIVE BRIDGE PLAY COMPLETE *Edwin B. Kantar*   10.00
____HOW TO IMPROVE YOUR BRIDGE *Alfred Sheinwold*   3.00
____IMPROVING YOUR BIDDING SKILLS *Edwin B. Kantar*   4.00
____INTRODUCTION TO DEFENDER'S PLAY *Edwin B. Kantar*   3.00
____SHORT CUT TO WINNING BRIDGE *Alfred Sheinwold*   3.00
____TEST YOUR BRIDGE PLAY *Edwin B. Kantar*   3.00
____WINNING DECLARER PLAY *Dorothy Hayden Truscott*   4.00

BUSINESS, STUDY & REFERENCE

____CONVERSATION MADE EASY *Elliot Russell*   2.00
____EXAM SECRET *Dennis B. Jackson*   3.00
____FIX-IT BOOK *Arthur Symons*   2.00
____HOW TO DEVELOP A BETTER SPEAKING VOICE *M. Hellier*   3.00
____HOW TO MAKE A FORTUNE IN REAL ESTATE *Albert Winnikoff*   4.00
____INCREASE YOUR LEARNING POWER *Geoffrey A. Dudley*   2.00
____MAGIC OF NUMBERS *Robert Tocquet*   2.00
____PRACTICAL GUIDE TO BETTER CONCENTRATION *Melvin Powers*   3.00
____PRACTICAL GUIDE TO PUBLIC SPEAKING *Maurice Forley*   3.00
____7 DAYS TO FASTER READING *William S. Schaill*   3.00
____SONGWRITERS RHYMING DICTIONARY *Jane Shaw Whitfield*   5.00
____SPELLING MADE EASY *Lester D. Basch & Dr. Milton Finkelstein*   2.00
____STUDENT'S GUIDE TO BETTER GRADES *J. A. Rickard*   3.00
____TEST YOURSELF—Find Your Hidden Talent *Jack Shafer*   3.00
____YOUR WILL & WHAT TO DO ABOUT IT *Attorney Samuel G. Kling*   3.00

CALLIGRAPHY

____ADVANCED CALLIGRAPHY *Katherine Jeffares*   7.00
____CALLIGRAPHER'S REFERENCE BOOK *Anne Leptich & Jacque Evans*   6.00
____CALLIGRAPHY—The Art of Beautiful Writing *Katherine Jeffares*   7.00
____CALLIGRAPHY FOR FUN & PROFIT *Anne Leptich & Jacque Evans*   7.00
____CALLIGRAPHY MADE EASY *Tina Serafini*   7.00

CHESS & CHECKERS

____BEGINNER'S GUIDE TO WINNING CHESS *Fred Reinfeld*   3.00
____BETTER CHESS—How to Play *Fred Reinfeld*   2.00
____CHECKERS MADE EASY *Tom Wiswell*   2.00
____CHESS IN TEN EASY LESSONS *Larry Evans*   3.00
____CHESS MADE EASY *Milton L. Hanauer*   3.00
____CHESS PROBLEMS FOR BEGINNERS *edited by Fred Reinfeld*   2.00
____CHESS SECRETS REVEALED *Fred Reinfeld*   2.00
____CHESS STRATEGY—An Expert's Guide *Fred Reinfeld*   2.00
____CHESS TACTICS FOR BEGINNERS *edited by Fred Reinfeld*   3.00
____CHESS THEORY & PRACTICE *Morry & Mitchell*   2.00
____HOW TO WIN AT CHECKERS *Fred Reinfeld*   3.00
____1001 BRILLIANT WAYS TO CHECKMATE *Fred Reinfeld*   3.00
____1001 WINNING CHESS SACRIFICES & COMBINATIONS *Fred Reinfeld*   4.00
____SOVIET CHESS *Edited by R. G. Wade*   3.00

COOKERY & HERBS

CULPEPER'S HERBAL REMEDIES *Dr. Nicholas Culpeper* — 3.00
FAST GOURMET COOKBOOK *Poppy Cannon* — 2.50
GINSENG The Myth & The Truth *Joseph P. Hou* — 3.00
HEALING POWER OF HERBS *May Bethel* — 3.00
HEALING POWER OF NATURAL FOODS *May Bethel* — 3.00
HERB HANDBOOK *Dawn MacLeod* — 3.00
HERBS FOR COOKING AND HEALING *Dr. Donald Law* — 2.00
HERBS FOR HEALTH—How to Grow & Use Them *Louise Evans Doole* — 3.00
HOME GARDEN COOKBOOK—Delicious Natural Food Recipes *Ken Kraft* — 3.00
MEDICAL HERBALIST *edited by Dr. J. R. Yemm* — 3.00
NATURAL FOOD COOKBOOK *Dr. Harry C. Bond* — 3.00
NATURE'S MEDICINES *Richard Lucas* — 3.00
VEGETABLE GARDENING FOR BEGINNERS *Hugh Wiberg* — 2.00
VEGETABLES FOR TODAY'S GARDENS *R. Milton Carleton* — 2.00
VEGETARIAN COOKERY *Janet Walker* — 4.00
VEGETARIAN COOKING MADE EASY & DELECTABLE *Veronica Vezza* — 3.00
VEGETARIAN DELIGHTS—A Happy Cookbook for Health *K. R. Mehta* — 2.00
VEGETARIAN GOURMET COOKBOOK *Joyce McKinnel* — 3.00

GAMBLING & POKER

ADVANCED POKER STRATEGY & WINNING PLAY *A. D. Livingston* — 3.00
HOW NOT TO LOSE AT POKER *Jeffrey Lloyd Castle* — 3.00
HOW TO WIN AT DICE GAMES *Skip Frey* — 3.00
HOW TO WIN AT POKER *Terence Reese & Anthony T. Watkins* — 3.00
SECRETS OF WINNING POKER *George S. Coffin* — 3.00
WINNING AT CRAPS *Dr. Lloyd T. Commins* — 3.00
WINNING AT GIN *Chester Wander & Cy Rice* — 3.00
WINNING AT POKER—An Expert's Guide *John Archer* — 3.00
WINNING AT 21—An Expert's Guide *John Archer* — 4.00
WINNING POKER SYSTEMS *Norman Zadeh* — 3.00

HEALTH

BEE POLLEN *Lynda Lyngheim & Jack Scagnetti* — 3.00
DR. LINDNER'S SPECIAL WEIGHT CONTROL METHOD *P. G. Lindner, M.D.* — 1.50
HELP YOURSELF TO BETTER SIGHT *Margaret Darst Corbett* — 0.00
HOW TO IMPROVE YOUR VISION *Dr. Robert A. Kraskin* — 3.00
HOW YOU CAN STOP SMOKING PERMANENTLY *Ernest Caldwell* — 3.00
MIND OVER PLATTER *Peter G. Lindner, M.D.* — 3.00
NATURE'S WAY TO NUTRITION & VIBRANT HEALTH *Robert J. Scrutton* — 3.00
NEW CARBOHYDRATE DIET COUNTER *Patti Lopez-Pereira* — 1.50
QUICK & EASY EXERCISES FOR FACIAL BEAUTY *Judy Smith-deal* — 2.00
QUICK & EASY EXERCISES FOR FIGURE BEAUTY *Judy Smith-deal* — 2.00
REFLEXOLOGY *Dr. Maybelle Segal* — 3.00
REFLEXOLOGY FOR GOOD HEALTH *Anna Kaye & Don C. Matchan* — 3.00
YOU CAN LEARN TO RELAX *Dr. Samuel Gutwirth* — 3.00
YOUR ALLERGY—What To Do About It *Allan Knight, M.D.* — 3.00

HOBBIES

BEACHCOMBING FOR BEGINNERS *Norman Hickin* — 2.00
BLACKSTONE'S MODERN CARD TRICKS *Harry Blackstone* — 3.00
BLACKSTONE'S SECRETS OF MAGIC *Harry Blackstone* — 3.00
COIN COLLECTING FOR BEGINNERS *Burton Hobson & Fred Reinfeld* — 2.00
ENTERTAINING WITH ESP *Tony 'Doc' Shiels* — 2.00
400 FASCINATING MAGIC TRICKS YOU CAN DO *Howard Thurston* — 3.00
HOW I TURN JUNK INTO FUN AND PROFIT *Sari* — 3.00
HOW TO PLAY THE HARMONICA FOR FUN & PROFIT *Hal Leighton* — 3.00
HOW TO WRITE A HIT SONG & SELL IT *Tommy Boyce* — 7.00
JUGGLING MADE EASY *Rudolf Dittrich* — 2.00
MAGIC MADE EASY *Byron Wels* — 2.00
STAMP COLLECTING FOR BEGINNERS *Burton Hobson* — 2.00

HORSE PLAYERS' WINNING GUIDES

BETTING HORSES TO WIN *Les Conklin* — 3.00
ELIMINATE THE LOSERS *Bob McKnight* — 3.00

HOW TO PICK WINNING HORSES *Bob McKnight*	3.00
HOW TO WIN AT THE RACES *Sam (The Genius) Lewin*	3.00
HOW YOU CAN BEAT THE RACES *Jack Kavanagh*	3.00
MAKING MONEY AT THE RACES *David Barr*	3.00
PAYDAY AT THE RACES *Les Conklin*	3.00
SMART HANDICAPPING MADE EASY *William Bauman*	3.00
SUCCESS AT THE HARNESS RACES *Barry Meadow*	3.00
WINNING AT THE HARNESS RACES—An Expert's Guide *Nick Cammarano*	3.00

HUMOR

HOW TO BE A COMEDIAN FOR FUN & PROFIT *King & Laufer*	2.00
HOW TO FLATTEN YOUR TUSH *Coach Marge Reardon*	2.00
JOKE TELLER'S HANDBOOK *Bob Orben*	3.00
JOKES FOR ALL OCCASIONS *Al Schock*	3.00
2000 NEW LAUGHS FOR SPEAKERS *Bob Orben*	3.00
2,500 JOKES TO START 'EM LAUGHING *Bob Orben*	3.00

HYPNOTISM

ADVANCED TECHNIQUES OF HYPNOSIS *Melvin Powers*	2.00
BRAINWASHING AND THE CULTS *Paul A. Verdier, Ph.D.*	3.00
CHILDBIRTH WITH HYPNOSIS *William S. Kroger, M.D.*	3.00
HOW TO SOLVE Your Sex Problems with Self-Hypnosis *Frank S. Caprio, M.D.*	3.00
HOW TO STOP SMOKING THRU SELF-HYPNOSIS *Leslie M. LeCron*	3.00
HOW TO USE AUTO-SUGGESTION EFFECTIVELY *John Duckworth*	3.00
HOW YOU CAN BOWL BETTER USING SELF-HYPNOSIS *Jack Heise*	3.00
HOW YOU CAN PLAY BETTER GOLF USING SELF-HYPNOSIS *Jack Heise*	3.00
HYPNOSIS AND SELF-HYPNOSIS *Bernard Hollander, M.D.*	3.00
HYPNOTISM *(Originally published in 1893) Carl Sextus*	5.00
HYPNOTISM & PSYCHIC PHENOMENA *Simeon Edmunds*	4.00
HYPNOTISM MADE EASY *Dr. Ralph Winn*	3.00
HYPNOTISM MADE PRACTICAL *Louis Orton*	3.00
HYPNOTISM REVEALED *Melvin Powers*	2.00
HYPNOTISM TODAY *Leslie LeCron and Jean Bordeaux, Ph.D.*	5.00
MODERN HYPNOSIS *Lesley Kuhn & Salvatore Russo, Ph.D.*	5.00
NEW CONCEPTS OF HYPNOSIS *Bernard C. Gindes, M.D.*	5.00
NEW SELF-HYPNOSIS *Paul Adams*	4.00
POST-HYPNOTIC INSTRUCTIONS—Suggestions for Therapy *Arnold Furst*	3.00
PRACTICAL GUIDE TO SELF-HYPNOSIS *Melvin Powers*	3.00
PRACTICAL HYPNOTISM *Philip Magonet, M.D.*	3.00
SECRETS OF HYPNOTISM *S. J. Van Pelt, M.D.*	3.00
SELF-HYPNOSIS A Conditioned-Response Technique *Laurance Sparks*	5.00
SELF-HYPNOSIS Its Theory, Technique & Application *Melvin Powers*	3.00
THERAPY THROUGH HYPNOSIS *edited by Raphael H. Rhodes*	4.00

JUDAICA

HOW TO LIVE A RICHER & FULLER LIFE *Rabbi Edgar F. Magnin*	2.00
MODERN ISRAEL *Lily Edelman*	2.00
SERVICE OF THE HEART *Evelyn Garfiel, Ph.D.*	4.00
STORY OF ISRAEL IN COINS *Jean & Maurice Gould*	2.00
STORY OF ISRAEL IN STAMPS *Maxim & Gabriel Shamir*	1.00

JUST FOR WOMEN

COSMOPOLITAN'S GUIDE TO MARVELOUS MEN Fwd. by *Helen Gurley Brown*	3.00
COSMOPOLITAN'S HANG-UP HANDBOOK Foreword by *Helen Gurley Brown*	4.00
COSMOPOLITAN'S LOVE BOOK—A Guide to Ecstasy in Bed	4.00
COSMOPOLITAN'S NEW ETIQUETTE GUIDE Fwd. by *Helen Gurley Brown*	4.00
I AM A COMPLEAT WOMAN *Doris Hagopian & Karen O'Connor Sweeney*	3.00
JUST FOR WOMEN—A Guide to the Female Body *Richard E. Sand, M.D.*	4.00
NEW APPROACHES TO SEX IN MARRIAGE *John E. Eichenlaub, M.D.*	3.00
SEXUALLY ADEQUATE FEMALE *Frank S. Caprio, M.D.*	3.00
YOUR FIRST YEAR OF MARRIAGE *Dr. Tom McGinnis*	3.00

MARRIAGE, SEX & PARENTHOOD

ABILITY TO LOVE *Dr. Allan Fromme*	5.00
ENCYCLOPEDIA OF MODERN SEX & LOVE TECHNIQUES *Macandrew*	5.00
GUIDE TO SUCCESSFUL MARRIAGE *Drs. Albert Ellis & Robert Harper*	5.00

HOW TO RAISE AN EMOTIONALLY HEALTHY, HAPPY CHILD *A. Ellis*	3.00
IMPOTENCE & FRIGIDITY *Edwin W. Hirsch, M.D.*	3.00
SEX WITHOUT GUILT *Albert Ellis, Ph.D.*	3.00
SEXUALLY ADEQUATE MALE *Frank S. Caprio, M.D.*	3.00

MELVIN POWERS' MAIL ORDER LIBRARY

HOW TO GET RICH IN MAIL ORDER *Melvin Powers*	10.00
HOW TO WRITE A GOOD ADVERTISEMENT *Victor O. Schwab*	15.00
WORLD WIDE MAIL ORDER SHOPPER'S GUIDE *Eugene V. Moller*	5.00

METAPHYSICS & OCCULT

BOOK OF TALISMANS, AMULETS & ZODIACAL GEMS *William Pavitt*	4.00
CONCENTRATION—A Guide to Mental Mastery *Mouni Sadhu*	3.00
CRITIQUES OF GOD *Edited by Peter Angeles*	7.00
DREAMS & OMENS REVEALED *Fred Gettings*	3.00
EXTRA-TERRESTRIAL INTELLIGENCE—The First Encounter	6.00
FORTUNE TELLING WITH CARDS *P. Foli*	3.00
HANDWRITING ANALYSIS MADE EASY *John Marley*	3.00
HANDWRITING TELLS *Nadya Olyanova*	5.00
HOW TO UNDERSTAND YOUR DREAMS *Geoffrey A. Dudley*	3.00
ILLUSTRATED YOGA *William Zorn*	3.00
IN DAYS OF GREAT PEACE *Mouni Sadhu*	3.00
KING SOLOMON'S TEMPLE IN THE MASONIC TRADITION *Alex Horne*	5.00
LSD—THE AGE OF MIND *Bernard Roseman*	2.00
MAGICIAN—His training and work *W. E. Butler*	3.00
MEDITATION *Mouni Sadhu*	5.00
MODERN NUMEROLOGY *Morris C. Goodman*	3.00
NUMEROLOGY—ITS FACTS AND SECRETS *Ariel Yvon Taylor*	3.00
NUMEROLOGY MADE EASY *W. Mykian*	3.00
PALMISTRY MADE EASY *Fred Gettings*	3.00
PALMISTRY MADE PRACTICAL *Elizabeth Daniels Squire*	3.00
PALMISTRY SECRETS REVEALED *Henry Frith*	3.00
PROPHECY IN OUR TIME *Martin Ebon*	2.50
PSYCHOLOGY OF HANDWRITING *Nadya Olyanova*	3.00
SUPERSTITION—Are you superstitious? *Eric Maple*	2.00
TAROT *Mouni Sadhu*	6.00
TAROT OF THE BOHEMIANS *Papus*	5.00
WAYS TO SELF-REALIZATION *Mouni Sadhu*	3.00
WHAT YOUR HANDWRITING REVEALS *Albert E. Hughes*	2.00
WITCHCRAFT, MAGIC & OCCULTISM—A Fascinating History *W. B. Crow*	5.00
WITCHCRAFT—THE SIXTH SENSE *Justine Glass*	4.00
WORLD OF PSYCHIC RESEARCH *Hereward Carrington*	2.00

SELF-HELP & INSPIRATIONAL

DAILY POWER FOR JOYFUL LIVING *Dr. Donald Curtis*	3.00
DYNAMIC THINKING *Melvin Powers*	2.00
EXUBERANCE—Your Guide to Happiness & Fulfillment *Dr. Paul Kurtz*	3.00
GREATEST POWER IN THE UNIVERSE *U. S. Andersen*	5.00
GROW RICH WHILE YOU SLEEP *Ben Sweetland*	3.00
GROWTH THROUGH REASON *Albert Ellis, Ph.D.*	4.00
GUIDE TO DEVELOPING YOUR POTENTIAL *Herbert A. Otto, Ph.D.*	3.00
GUIDE TO LIVING IN BALANCE *Frank S. Caprio, M.D.*	2.00
HELPING YOURSELF WITH APPLIED PSYCHOLOGY *R. Henderson*	2.00
HELPING YOURSELF WITH PSYCHIATRY *Frank S. Caprio, M.D.*	2.00
HOW TO ATTRACT GOOD LUCK *A. H. Z. Carr*	4.00
HOW TO CONTROL YOUR DESTINY *Norvell*	3.00
HOW TO DEVELOP A WINNING PERSONALITY *Martin Panzer*	3.00
HOW TO DEVELOP AN EXCEPTIONAL MEMORY *Young & Gibson*	4.00
HOW TO OVERCOME YOUR FEARS *M. P. Leahy, M.D.*	3.00
HOW YOU CAN HAVE CONFIDENCE AND POWER *Les Giblin*	3.00
HUMAN PROBLEMS & HOW TO SOLVE THEM *Dr. Donald Curtis*	3.00
I CAN *Ben Sweetland*	4.00
I WILL *Ben Sweetland*	3.00
LEFT-HANDED PEOPLE *Michael Barsley*	4.00

*The books listed above can be obtained from your book dealer or directly from
Melvin Powers. When ordering, please remit 50¢ per book postage & handling.
Send for our free illustrated catalog of self-improvement books.*

Melvin Powers

12015 Sherman Road, No. Hollywood, California 91605